T0202640

Communications
in Computer and Information Science 2080

Editorial Board Members

Rationale

The CCIS series is devoted to the publication of proceedings of computer science conferences. Its aim is to efficiently disseminate original research results in informatics in printed and electronic form. While the focus is on publication of peer-reviewed full papers presenting mature work, inclusion of reviewed short papers reporting on work in progress is welcome, too. Besides globally relevant meetings with internationally representative program committees guaranteeing a strict peer-reviewing and paper selection process, conferences run by societies or of high regional or national relevance are also considered for publication.

Topics

The topical scope of CCIS spans the entire spectrum of informatics ranging from foundational topics in the theory of computing to information and communications science and technology and a broad variety of interdisciplinary application fields.

Information for Volume Editors and Authors

Publication in CCIS is free of charge. No royalties are paid, however, we offer registered conference participants temporary free access to the online version of the conference proceedings on SpringerLink (http://link.springer.com) by means of an http referrer from the conference website and/or a number of complimentary printed copies, as specified in the official acceptance email of the event.

CCIS proceedings can be published in time for distribution at conferences or as post-proceedings, and delivered in the form of printed books and/or electronically as USBs and/or e-content licenses for accessing proceedings at SpringerLink. Furthermore, CCIS proceedings are included in the CCIS electronic book series hosted in the SpringerLink digital library at http://link.springer.com/bookseries/7899. Conferences publishing in CCIS are allowed to use Online Conference Service (OCS) for managing the whole proceedings lifecycle (from submission and reviewing to preparing for publication) free of charge.

Publication process

The language of publication is exclusively English. Authors publishing in CCIS have to sign the Springer CCIS copyright transfer form, however, they are free to use their material published in CCIS for substantially changed, more elaborate subsequent publications elsewhere. For the preparation of the camera-ready papers/files, authors have to strictly adhere to the Springer CCIS Authors' Instructions and are strongly encouraged to use the CCIS LaTeX style files or templates.

Abstracting/Indexing

CCIS is abstracted/indexed in DBLP, Google Scholar, EI-Compendex, Mathematical Reviews, SCImago, Scopus. CCIS volumes are also submitted for the inclusion in ISI Proceedings.

How to start

To start the evaluation of your proposal for inclusion in the CCIS series, please send an e-mail to ccis@springer.com.

Hua Xu · Qingcai Chen · Hongfei Lin · Fei Wu ·
Lei Liu · Buzhou Tang · Tianyong Hao ·
Zhengxing Huang · Jianbo Lei · Zuofeng Li ·
Hui Zong

Editors

Health Information Processing

Evaluation Track Papers

9th China Conference, CHIP 2023
Hangzhou, China, October 27–29, 2023
Proceedings

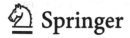 Springer

Editors
Hua Xu
The University of Texas Health Science
Center at Houston
Houston, TX, USA

Hongfei Lin ⓘ
Dalian University of Technology
Dalian, China

Lei Liu
Fudan University
Shanghai, China

Tianyong Hao ⓘ
South China Normal University
Guangzhou, China

Jianbo Lei ⓘ
Medical Informatics Center of Peking
University
Beijing, China

Hui Zong ⓘ
West China Hospital of Sichuan University
Chengdu, China

Qingcai Chen ⓘ
Harbin Institute of Technology
Shenzhen, China

Fei Wu
Zhejiang University
Hangzhou, China

Buzhou Tang ⓘ
Harbin Institute of Technology
Shenzhen, China

Zhengxing Huang ⓘ
Zhejiang University
Hangzhou, China

Zuofeng Li ⓘ
Takeda Co. Ltd
Shanghai, China

ISSN 1865-0929   ISSN 1865-0937 (electronic)
Communications in Computer and Information Science
ISBN 978-981-97-1716-3   ISBN 978-981-97-1717-0 (eBook)
https://doi.org/10.1007/978-981-97-1717-0

This Springer imprint is published by the registered company Springer Nature Singapore Pte Ltd.
The registered company address is: 152 Beach Road, #21-01/04 Gateway East, Singapore 189721, Singapore

Paper in this product is recyclable.

Preface

Health information processing and applications is an essential field in data-driven health and clinical medicine and it has been highly active in recent decades. The China Health Information Processing Conference (CHIP) is an annual conference held by the Medical Health and Biological Information Processing Committee of the Chinese Information Processing Society (CIPS) of China, with the theme of "large models and smart health-care". CHIP is one of the leading conferences in the field of health information processing in China and turned into an international event in 2023. It is also an important platform for researchers and practitioners from academia, business and government departments around the world to share ideas and further promote research and applications in this field. CHIP 2023 was organized by Zhejiang University and was held in hybrid online/offline format, whereby people could attend face-to-face or freely connect to live broadcasts of keynote speeches and presentations.

CHIP 2023 Evaluation released 6 shared tasks, including CHIP-PromptCBLUE Medical Large Model Evaluation Task, Chinese Medical Text Few-Shot Named Entity Recognition Evaluation Task, Drug Paper Document Recognition and Entity Relation Extraction Task, CHIP-YIER Medical Large Model Evaluation Task, Medical Literature PICOS Identification Task and Chinese Diabetes Question Classification Task. Hundreds of teams from both academia and industry participated in the shared tasks. A total of 15 high-ranking teams were selected to submit algorithm papers. The organizer of the shared tasks also submitted 6 overview papers. The 21 papers included in this volume were carefully chosen for publication after a single-blind peer review process, with an average of 1.33 reviewers assigned to each submission.

The authors of each paper in this volume reported their novel results, computing methods or applications. The volume cannot cover all aspects of Medical Health and Biological Information Processing but may still inspire insightful thoughts for the readers. We hope that more secrets of Health Information Processing will be unveiled, and that academics will drive more practical developments and solutions.

November 2023

Hua Xu
Qingcai Chen
Hongfei Lin
Fei Wu
Lei Liu
Buzhou Tang
Tianyong Hao
Zhengxing Huang
Jianbo Lei
Zuofeng Li
Hui Zong

Organization

Honorary Chairs

Hua Xu   UTHealth, USA
Qingcai Chen   Harbin Institute of Technology (Shenzhen), China

General Co-chairs

Hongfei Lin   Dalian University of Technology, China
Fei Wu   Zhejiang University, China
Lei Liu   Fudan University, China

Program Co-chairs

Buzhou Tang   Harbin Institute of Technology (Shenzhen) &
                             Pengcheng Laboratory, China
Tianyong Hao   South China Normal University, China
Yanshan Wang   University of Pittsburgh, USA
Maggie Haitian Wang   Chinese University of Hong Kong, China

Young Scientists Forum Co-chairs

Zhengxing Huang   Zhejiang University, China
Yonghui Wu   University of Florida, USA

Publication Co-chairs

Fengfeng Zhou   Jilin University, China
Yongjun Zhu   Yonsei University, South Korea

Evaluation Co-chairs

Jianbo Lei   Medical Informatics Center of Peking University,
                                  China
Zuofeng Li   Takeda Co. Ltd, China

Publicity Co-chairs

Siwei Yu   Guizhou Medical University, China
Lishuang Li   Dalian University of Technology, China

Sponsor Co-chairs

Jun Yan   Yidu Cloud (Beijing) Technology Co., Ltd. China
Buzhou Tang   Harbin Institute of Technology (Shenzhen) &
                                  Pengcheng Laboratory, China

Web Chair

Kunli Zhang   Zhengzhou University, China

Program Committee

Wenping Guo   Taizhou University, China
Hongmin Cai   South China University of Technology, China
Chao Che   Dalian University, China
Mosha Chen   Alibaba, China
Qingcai Chen   Harbin Institute of Technology (Shenzhen), China
Xi Chen   Tencent Technology Co., Ltd, China
Yang Chen   Yidu Cloud (Beijing) Technology Co., Ltd, China
Zhumin Chen   Shandong University, China
Ming Cheng   Zhengzhou University, China
Ruoyao Ding   Guangdong University of Foreign Studies, China
Bin Dong   Ricoh Software Research Center (Beijing) Co.,
                                  Ltd, China
Guohong Fu   Soochow University, China
Yan Gao   Central South University, China
Tianyong Hao   South China Normal University, China

Shizhu He	Institute of Automation, Chinese Academy of Sciences, China
Zengyou He	Dalian University of Technology, China
Na Hong	Digital China Medical Technology Co., Ltd, China
Li Hou	Institute of Medical Information, Chinese Academy of Medical Sciences, China
Yong Hu	Jinan University, China
Baotian Hu	Harbin University of Technology (Shenzhen), China
Guimin Huang	Guilin University of Electronic Science and Technology, China
Zhenghang Huang	Zhejiang University, China
Zhiwei Huang	Southwest Medical University, China
Bo Jin	Dalian University of Technology, China
Xiaoyu Kang	Southwest Medical University, China
Jianbo Lei	Peking University, China
Haomin Li	Children's Hospital of Zhejiang University Medical College, China
Jiao Li	Institute of Medical Information, Chinese Academy of Medical Sciences, China
Jinghua Li	Chinese Academy of Traditional Chinese Medicine, China
Lishuang Li	Dalian University of Technology, China
Linfeng Li	Yidu Cloud (Beijing) Technology Co., Ltd, China
Ru Li	Shanxi University, China
Runzhi Li	Zhengzhou University, China
Shasha Li	National University of Defense Technology, China
Xing Li	Beijing Shenzhengyao Technology Co., Ltd, China
Xin Li	Zhongkang Physical Examination Technology Co., Ltd, China
Yuxi Li	Peking University First Hospital, China
Zuofeng Li	Takeda China, China
Xiangwen Liao	Fuzhou University, China
Hao Lin	University of Electronic Science and Technology of China, China
Hongfei Lin	Dalian University of Technology, China
Bangtao Liu	Southwest Medical University, China
Song Liu	Qilu University of Technology, China
Lei Liu	Fudan University, China
Shengping Liu	Unisound Co., Ltd, China

Xiaoming Liu	Zhongyuan University of Technology, China
Guan Luo	Institute of Automation, Chinese Academy of Sciences, China
Lingyun Luo	Nanhua University, China
Yamei Luo	Southwest Medical University, China
Hui Lv	Shanghai Jiaotong University, China
Xudong Lv	Zhejiang University, China
Yao Meng	Lenovo Research Institute, China
Qingliang Miao	AISpeech Co., Ltd, China
Weihua Peng	Baidu Co., Ltd, China
Buyue Qian	Xi'an Jiaotong University, China
Longhua Qian	Suzhou University, China
Tong Ruan	East China University of Technology, China
Ying Shen	South China University of Technology, China
Xiaofeng Song	Nanjing University of Aeronautics and Astronautics, China
Chengjie Sun	Harbin University of Technology, China
Chuanji Tan	Alibaba Dharma Hall, China
Hongye Tan	Shanxi University, China
Jingyu Tan	Shenzhen Xinkaiyuan Information Technology Development Co., Ltd, China
Binhua Tang	Hehai University, China
Buzhou Tang	Harbin Institute of Technology (Shenzhen), China
Jintao Tang	National Defense University of the People's Liberation Army, China
Qian Tao	South China University of Technology, China
Fei Teng	Southwest Jiaotong University, China
Shengwei Tian	Xinjiang University, China
Dong Wang	Southern Medical University, China
Haitian Wang	Chinese University of Hong Kong, China
Haofen Wang	Tongji University, China
Xiaolei Wang	Hong Kong Institute of Sustainable Development Education, China
Haolin Wang	Chongqing Medical University, China
Yehan Wang	Unisound AI Technology Co., Ltd, China
Zhenyu Wang	South China Institute of Technology Software, China
Zhongmin Wang	Jiangsu Provincial People's Hospital, China
Leyi Wei	Shandong University, China
Heng Weng	Guangdong Hospital of Traditional Chinese Medicine, China
Gang Wu	Beijing Knowledge Atlas Technology Co., Ltd, China

Xian Wu	Tencent Technology (Beijing) Co., Ltd, China
Jingbo Xia	Huazhong Agricultural University, China
Lu Xiang	Institute of Automation, Chinese Academy of Sciences, China
Yang Xiang	Pengcheng Laboratory, China
Lei Xu	Shenzhen Polytechnic, China
Liang Xu	Ping An Technology (Shenzhen) Co., Ltd, China
Yan Xu	Beihang University, Microsoft Asia Research Institute, China
Jun Yan	Yidu Cloud (Beijing) Technology Co., Ltd, China
Cheng Yang	Institute of Automation, Chinese Academy of Sciences, China
Hai Yang	East China University of Technology, China
Meijie Yang	Chongqing Medical University, China
Muyun Yang	Harbin University of Technology, China
Zhihao Yang	Dalian University of Technology, China
Hui Ye	Guangzhou University of Traditional Chinese Medicine, China
Dehui Yin	Southwest Medical University, China
Qing Yu	Xinjiang University, China
Liang Yu	Xi'an University of Electronic Science and Technology, China
Siwei Yu	Guizhou Provincial People's Hospital, China
Hongying Zan	Zhengzhou University, China
Hao Zhang	Jilin University, China
Kunli Zhang	Zhengzhou University, China
Weide Zhang	Zhongshan Hospital Affiliated to Fudan University, China
Xiaoyan Zhang	Tongji University, China
Yaoyun Zhang	Alibaba, China
Yijia Zhang	Dalian University of Technology, China
Yuanzhe Zhang	Institute of Automation, Chinese Academy of Sciences, China
Zhichang Zhang	Northwest Normal University, China
Qiuye Zhao	Beijing Big Data Research Institute, China
Sendong Zhao	Harbin Institute of Technology, China
Tiejun Zhao	Harbin Institute of Technology, China
Deyu Zhou	Southeast University, China
Fengfeng Zhou	Jilin University, China
Guangyou Zhou	Central China Normal University, China
Yi Zhou	Sun Yat-sen University, China
Conghui Zhu	Harbin Institute of Technology, China
Shanfeng Zhu	Fudan University, China

Yu Zhu	Sunshine Life Insurance Co., Ltd, China
Quan Zou	University of Electronic Science and Technology of China, China
Xi Chen	University of Electronic Science and Technology of China, China
Yansheng Li	Mediway Technology Co., Ltd, China
Daojing He	Harbin Institute of Technology (Shenzhen), China
Yupeng Liu	Harbin University of Science and Technology, China
Xinzhi Sun	First Affiliated Hospital of Zhengzhou University, China
Chuanchao Du	Third People's Hospital of Henan Province, China
Xien Liu	Beijing Huijizhiyi Technology Co., Ltd, China
Shan Nan	Hainan University, China
Xinyu He	Liaoning Normal University, China
Qianqian He	Chongqing Medical University, China
Xing Liu	Third Xiangya Hospital of Central South University, China
Jiayin Wang	Xi'an Jiaotong University, China
Ying Xu	Xi'an Jiaotong University, China
Xin Lai	Xi'an Jiaotong University, China

Contents

Chinese Diabetes Question Classification

CHIP-PromptCBLUE Medical Large Model Evaluation

Overview of the PromptCBLUE Shared Task in CHIP2023

Wei Zhu[1]([✉]), Xiaoling Wang[1], Mosha Chen[2], and Buzhou Tang[3]

[1] East China Normal University, Shanghai, China
wzhu@stu.ecnu.edu.cn
[2] Holoflow Digital Technology, Hangzhou, China
[3] Harbin Institute of Technology, Shenzhen, China

Abstract. This paper presents an overview of the PromptCBLUE shared task (http://cips-chip.org.cn/2023/eval1) held in the CHIP-2023 Conference. This shared task reformulates the CBLUE benchmark, and provide a good testbed for Chinese open-domain or medical-domain large language models (LLMs) in general medical natural language processing. Two different tracks are held: (a) prompt tuning track, investigating the multitask prompt tuning of LLMs, (b) probing the in-context learning capabilities of open-sourced LLMs. Many teams from both the industry and academia participated in the shared tasks, and the top teams achieved amazing test results. This paper describes the tasks, the datasets, evaluation metrics, and the top systems for both tasks. Finally, the paper summarizes the techniques and results of the evaluation of the various approaches explored by the participating teams.

Keywords: PromptCBLUE · Large language models · Medical natural language processing · parameter efficient fine-tuning · in-context learning

1 Introduction

In 2023, the launch of large language models like ChatGPT, gpt-4, Claude, Bard have taken the world by surprise. People are amazed by their general capabilities: (a) universal NLP task solver [39]. (b) powerful chatting capabilities. (c) following human instructions [3,36]. (d) reasoning and planning capabilities [49]. Recent works have shown that these powerful LLMs have expert level knowledge in the medical domain [44]. Although these models are powerful, they are proprietary, and can not be deployed locally, preventing many applications that have serious privacy concerns [53]. Recently, more and more powerful open-sourced LLMs are being released [31], making it more and more convenient for developers to train or fine-tune a local LLM for application developments.

In order to evaluate the multitask capabilities of the recent open-sourced Chinese LLMs in medical NLP tasks, we re-build the CBLUE benchmark [57] into PromptCBLUE [76], a large-scale multi-task prompt tuning benchmark dataset (see Fig. 1). This benchmark is one of first and largest prompt tuning benchmark for medical LLMs in Chinese. The PromptCBLUE shared task is held in

H. Xu et al. (Eds.): CHIP 2023, CCIS 2080, pp. 3–20, 2024.
https://doi.org/10.1007/978-981-97-1717-0_1

the 2023 China Health Information Processing Conference, with the help of the conference committees. The shared task evaluate Chinese LLMs in two aspects, corresponding to two tracks: (a) the Parameter-efficient Fine-tuning (PEFT) Track, and (b) the In-Context Learning (ICL) Track.

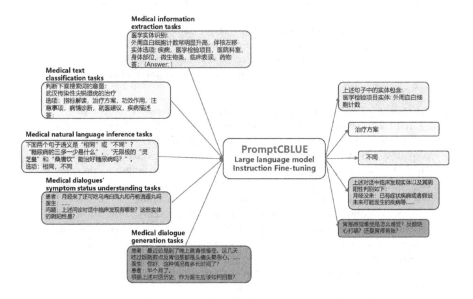

Fig. 1. We introduce PromptCBLUE, a large-scale instruction tuning benchmark for Chinese medical LLMs, which converts different types of medical natural language processing tasks into a unified prompt-response generation task. PromptCBLUE consists of five cohorts of 18 tasks, which cover a variety of medical applications.

The PEFT track is closely related to the recent trend of PEFT in the LLM research. Despite LLMs becoming general task solvers, fine-tuning still plays a vital role in efficient LLM inference and controlling the style of the LLMs' generated contents.[1] Fine-tuning such large models by full parameters is prohibitive since it requires a large amount of GPU memory and computations. Thus, parameter-efficient fine-tuning (PEFT) [60,62] has raised much attention in the research field since in PEFT, the tunable parameters are often less than 1% of the LLMs and the computation costs will be significantly decreased. In the PEFT Track, participants are asked to fine-tune a given open-sourced Chinese LLM with a single PEFT module for all the 18 sub-tasks of PromptCBLUE, while keeping the backbone LLM unchanged. This track intends to challenge the participants to come up with novel PEFT modules or novel multi-task training methods.

---

[1] Recently, OpenAI also released the fine-tuning API for GPT-3.5-turbo. See blog post: https://openai.com/blog/gpt-3-5-turbo-fine-tuning-and-api-updates.

With the recent advancements in scaling up model parameters, large language models (LLMs) showcase promising results on a variety of few-shot tasks through in-context learning (ICL), where the model is expected to directly generate the output of the test sample without updating parameters. This is achieved by conditioning on a manually designed prompt consisting of an optional task description and a few demonstration examples [40]. Since then, many efforts have been made on ICL [22]. In the ICL Track of, participants are asked to push the limit of ICL for medium sized (6B, 7B or 13B parameters) open-sourced LLMs. The backbone LLMs are freezed and they are not allowed to introduce any additional parameters to the backbone models. However, they can improve the LLMs' performance by designing better prompts, especially select proper demonstrations for any given samples. A BERT base model or any model with a similar size is allowed to facilitate the demonstration selection.

The PromptCBLUE shared task has raised much attention in both the industry and academia. A total of 600 teams have participated in either track of the shared task, and 48 teams have submitted predictions for the second round. In this paper, we will review the shared task, the winning teams and their methodologies, and discuss future research directions.

2   Related Work

2.1   Medical Natural Language Processing

The developments in neural networks and natural language processing has advanced the field of medical natural language processing (MedNLP) [11,63–65,69,71,73]. In the pre-BERT era, firstly, RNNs like LSTM/GRU are used for processing sequential medical data such as text and speech [1]. Convolutional networks are also used for medical text classification [14,66]. The techniques of Graph neural networks are also explored for diagnose recommendations [24]. In this period, many different model architectures are specially designed for better performances on a specific MedNLP task [61,71,75]. Since BERT [6], the pretrained language models (PLMs) become the default solution for MedNLP. In this stage, researcher becomes less interested in modifying the model architecture, but instead trying to pretrain or further pretrain a PLM from the open domain to the medical domain [8,10,48,67,68].

With the wide study of LLMs, the field of MedNLP is also being revolutionized. There are already works on adapting LLM backbones to the medical domain question answering [74]. And [76] propose PromptCBLUE, a prompt learning based benchmark dataset for examining the LLMs' ability in MedNLP tasks. This work investigates the capabilities of both the commercial LLMs like ChatGPT, and the open-sourced ones by employing the PromptCBLUE as the testbed, providing a deeper understanding of LLMs for future MedNLP research.

2.2 Parameter-Efficient Fine-Tuning

In this subsection, we review currently the most popular PEFT methods.

Adapter-Based Tuning. One of the most important research lines of PEFT is adapter-based tuning. Adapter [13] inserts adapter modules with bottleneck architecture between every consecutive Transformer [46] sublayers. AdapterFusion [37] only inserts sequential adapters after the feed-forward module. Adapter-based tuning methods have comparable results with model tuning when only tuning a fraction of the backbone model's parameter number. Due to their strong performance, a branch of literature has investigated the architecture of adapters in search of further improvements. [12] analyze a wide range of PETuning methods and show that they are essentially equivalent. They also propose the general architecture of PEFT, and derive the Parallel Adapter which connects the adapter modules in parallel to the self-attention and MLP modules in the Transformer block. AdapterDrop [43] investigates the efficiency of removing adapters from lower layers. Adaptive adapters [35] investigate the activation functions of adapters and propose to learn the activation functions of adapters via optimizing the parameters of rational functions as a part of the model parameters. Compacter [33] uses low-rank parameterized hypercomplex multiplication [18] to compress adapters' tunable parameters. LST [45] improves the memory efficiency by forming the adapters as a ladder along stacked Transformer blocks, and it enhances the adapter module by adding a self-attention module to its bottleneck architecture. [15, 45, 59] try to add different encoding operations, like self-attention operations and convolutions between the bottleneck structure of adapters, and achieve better performances. Learned-Adapter [60] builds upon the above adapter-based methods and enhance the performance of adapter tuning by automatically learning better architectures for adapters.

Prompt Tuning Methods. Prompt tuning [19] and P-tuning [30] insert a soft prompt to word embeddings only, and can achieve competitive results when applied to supersized PTMs. Prefix-tuning [21] and P-tuning v2 [29] insert prompts to every hidden layer of PTM. IDPG [50] uses the prompt generator with parameterized hypercomplex multiplication [18] to generate a soft prompt for every instance. LPT [28] improves upon IDPG by selecting an intermediate layer to start inserting prompts. SPT [72] designs a mechanism to automatically decide which layers to insert new instance-aware soft prompts.

Literature for the LoRA Methods. Since LoRA is the most popular PEFT method in the era of large language models, there are many works that are orthogonal to AdaLoRA, SoRA and our work that are devoted to improve LoRA on many different aspects. QLoRA [5] proposes a novel quantization method that can significantly reduce the memory consumptions of LLMs during LoRA fine-tuning. LoRA-FA [56] freezes parts of the randomly initialized LoRA matrices. (d) VERA [17] investigate whether one could froze the randomly initialized LoRA matrices and only learns a set of scaling vectors. Tying LoRA matrices across layers are also investigated by VERA.

2.3   In-Context Learning

GPT-3 [40], the OpenAI's former SOTA LLM, raise the attention of the research field to a novel research direction: in-context learning (ICL). In their paper, they have showcased that GPT-3, a self-supervised pretrained model, can immediately master a new task it is never trained on by reading a manually designed prompt consisting of an optional task description and a few demonstration examples. Since then, a branch of literature has been devoted to investigate different aspects of ICL. A series of theoretical analysis attempted to understand why ICL works [4,16,34]. [4] explains language models as meta-optimizers and understand in-context learning as implicit fine-tuning. They prove that GPT first produces meta-gradients according to the demonstration examples, and then these meta-gradients are applied to the original GPT to build an ICL model. Since performance of ICL has been shown to be highly sensitive to the selection of demonstration examples [22]. [42] proposed to learn to retrieve demonstration examples. [22] proposes a series of techniques to enhance the performance of demonstration selection. [20] selected diverse demonstrations to improve in-context compositional generalization. More recent studies have explored leveraging the output distributions of language models to select few-shot demonstrations [23]. [38] iteratively selects examples that are diverse but still strongly correlated with the test sample as ICL demonstrations.

3   Overview of PromptCBLUE

3.1   Overview

Built upon the CBLUE benchmark [57], we created an extensive multi-task test suite in the medical domain for the LLMs that supports Chinese. The tasks in PromptCBLUE can be divided into the following groups:

- **Medical information extraction**, including: (a) CMeEE-V2 [54], a medical named entity recognition task. (b) CMeIE [9], a medical triple extraction task. (c) CHIP-CDEE, which asks models to extract clinical finding events; (d) CHIP-CDN, which asks one to map the diagnosis descriptions to standard ICD-10^2 disease terms. (e) IMCS-V2-NER for extracting medical entities in the dialogues from the medical dialogue datasets IMCS-V2 [2]. (f) Text2DT, which is a complex medical information extraction task proposed by [70]. This novel task asks a model to extract medical decision processes in the format of binary trees from the unstructured medical text. (g) CmedCausal [25], which asks a model to extract triplets with causal relations from unstructured medical documents.
- **Medical text classification**, which includes: (a) CHIP-CTC [77], the classification task for Chinese eligibility criteria in clinical trials. (b) KUAKE-QIC, which classifies online medical queries. (c) IMCS-V2-DAC for medical intent classification of medical dialogues.

---

^{2} https://www.whofic.nl/familie-van-internationale-classificaties/referentie-classificaties/icd-10.

- **Medical natural language inference tasks**, including CHIP-STS [32], KUAKE-QQR, KUAKE-IR, and KUAKE-QTR tasks, which asks a model to determine the semantic relations between a pair of medical queries or a query-document pair.
- **Symptom status understanding for medical dialogues**. Medical dialogues, like medical consultations, are centered around the patients' symptoms. However, not every symptom mentioned in the dialogues is related to patients or reflects patients' current medical status. Thus, to gain a deep understanding of the doctor-patient dialogues, a model must be able to extract the symptoms and their statuses. This cohort includes (a) IMCS-V2-SR and (b) CHIP-MDCFNPC for extracting clinical findings and their status. This cohort of tasks is based on the medical dialogue datasets IMCS-V2 [2] and CHIP-MDCFNPC [52].
- **Medical content generation**, which includes two generation tasks based on medical dialogues between patients and doctors: (a) IMCS-V2-MRG [2], which asks LLMs to summarize the medical dialogues. (b) MedDG [27], which asks LLMs to act like a doctor and respond to the patient's queries in a dialogue.

3.2   Prompt Collection

We employ both manual efforts and ChatGPT to collect prompt templates for PromptCBLUE. The prompt templates mainly contain task instructions describing what we want the LLMs to provide, given the text input. Firstly, each of the three annotators who are graduate students majoring in computer science and are studying LLMs will write around two seed prompt templates manually. We ask the annotators to write the prompts as diversified as possible. The prompt templates are then reviewed by a panel of two medical experts and a senior NLP researcher to ensure their validity. If a prompt is not proper (for example, not expressing the task clearly), we will ask the annotators to modify it until the domain experts accept it. Then, we will ask the ChatGPT to rephrase each of the six seed prompts templates ten times without changing the meaning or changing the placeholders in the templates. Then, the generated templates will be reviewed by the same panel of experts, and only the templates passing the reviews will be added to the template pool. After the prompt collection process, there are a total of 320 prompt templates in PromptCBLUE.[3]

3.3   Response Format

Note that LLMs can only generate token sequences to represent their answers to the queries. We have to transform the structured outputs of the original CBLUE tasks into natural language sequences. In the Appendix, we present the target output formats for each task under PromptCBLUE.

---

[3] The manually written prompt templates and the augmented template sets are open-sourced at our code repository, https://github.com/michael-wzhu/PromptCBLUE.

Recently, [47,49] show that LLMs' reasoning or task-solving ability can be improved if LLMs are asked to complete the task step-by-step or reason step-by-step, that is, chain-of-thought (COT) prompting. In this task, inspired by [49], we will explore the idea of COT in the design of prompt and response formats for complex medical information extraction tasks. Take CMeIE as an example. With COT, in the prompt, we will ask the LLM to determine the existing relations in the given sentence and then extract the triples for each relation. Accordingly, in the response, first, the relations will be presented, and then the extracted triples will be organized into relation groups. Without COT, the prompt will not instruct the LLM to solve the task step-by-step, and in the response, the triples will be generated one by one. In this work, unless stated otherwise, we will use the prompt and response formats with COT for the CMeEE-V2, CMeIE, CHIP-CDEE, and IMCS-V2-NER tasks. We will use ablation studies to demonstrate that COT benefits in-context learning of LLMs like ChatGPT and fine-tuned open-sourced LLMs.

3.4   Sample Format

In PromptCBLUE, all the samples from different tasks are organized in the following data structure:

```
{
  "input": str,
  "target": str,
  "answer_choices": Union[list, Nonetype],
  "sample_id": str,
  "task_type": str,
  "task_dataset": str,
}
```

Here, *input* is the prompt sequence, *target* is the response we want the model to output, or at least the model should generate responses that contain the answers to the prompt. The other four keys are auxiliary, and the LLMs will not use them. *sample_id* is the sample index. *answer_choices* is the label option allowed by the prompt. The value for this key will be *None* if the task does not have a predefined label set. *task_dataset* specifies the task name in the original CBLUE benchmark, and *task_type* is the original CBLUE task type.

3.5   Dataset Splits

Note that after filling in the CBLUE data samples in the prompt templates, the train/dev/test sets for some tasks will be quite large. Considering that LLMs require high computation resources to fine-tune and have large latency for token sequence generation, we limit the training samples of each task to 3000 to 5000 and the dev/test set to 400. We first fill each prompt template with the samples to construct a large test sample pool and randomly select the prompt-response

Table 1. Dataset statistics for the PromptCBLUE benchmark.

Task	#Train/#dev/#test	Prompt length	target length
Sub-tasks			
CMeEE-V2	5000/400/400	107.88	54.03
CMeIE	5000/400/400	293.72	135.51
CHIP-CDEE	3000/400/400	142.61	180.93
CHIP-CDN	5000/400/400	281.79	10.37
CHIP-CTC	6600/704/704	214.61	3.81
CHIP-STS	5000/400/400	66.26	2.0
KUAKE-QIC	5500/440/440	81.58	4.09
KUAKE-QTR	5000/400/400	96.38	7.23
KUAKE-QQR	5000/400/400	89.38	7.61
KUAKE-IR	5000/400/400	203.33	2.78
CHIP-MDCFNPC	5000/400/400	744.99	67.67
IMCS-V2-SR	5000/400/400	137.13	36.33
IMCS-V2-NER	5000/400/400	61.66	23.65
IMCS-V2-DAC	5000/512/512	371.62	8.56
IMCS-V2-MRG	3000/400/400	821.1	105.08
MedDG	5000/400/400	194.75	27.71
Text2DT	1500/400/400	465.10	392.47
CMedCausal	3000/400/400	423.68	272.25
Total			
PromptCBLUE	87100/8456/8456	265.22	71.10

pairs via uniform sampling.[4] In Table 1, we present the dataset statistics for the PromptCBLUE dataset.

Quality Checking. The quality check of our data is conducted in the following three aspects:

- Ensuring the quality of the prompt templates with the help of the expert panel, as described above.
- Checking the quality of the CBLUE benchmark. During the development of the PromptCBLUE benchmark, we are also helping the CBLUE benchmark to improve the annotations. For example, we have found that the original QQR task has an inappropriate label set and asked the CBLUE organizers to re-annotate this task.
- Random sampling. To ensure the data quality, we sampled 5% or 200 of the samples from each task of PromptCBLUE, and each sample was examined by

---

[4] Note that the training set is provided just as a reference for participants in the Tianchi competition since some of the original CBLUE tasks have large training sets.

a group of annotators from the medical field. Finally, we identify an average of 0.9% mislabeling rate. Based on the evaluation results in the next section, such an error rate will not significantly impact the overall evaluation accuracy.

3.6 Evaluation Metrics

Since metrics like BLUE or ROUGE [26] can not properly measure how LLMs perform for some of the PromptCBLUE tasks like medical information extraction tasks, we use post-processing scripts to transform the output sequences to structured data formats. PromptCBLUE adopts the following metrics:

- Instance-level strict micro-F1 for medical information extraction tasks, IMCS-V2-SR and CHIP-MDCFNPC. Here, an instance means a piece of complete information extracted from the given document. For example, in CMeEE-V2, an instance consists of an entity mention extracted and its predicted entity label. Furthermore, in IMCS-V2-SR, an instance consists of two keys: the entity mention of a symptom and its status. We adopt the strict metrics, meaning that the model predicts an instance correctly if and only if it correctly predicts all the keys of an instance.
- For medical text classification tasks and the IMCS-V2-DAC tasks, we adopt the macro-F1 score.
- For medical natural language inference tasks, we adopt the micro-F1 score.
- For the medical content generation tasks, we adopt ROUGE-L [26] as the metric.

4 Participating Teams and Methods

4.1 Participating Teams

This shared task is held in CHIP-2023 Conference as Shared Task 1. We held this shared task with the help the Tianchi Team, and all the logistics are handled by the Tianchi platform.[5] In the first round of the shared task, 362 teams participated in the PEFT track, and 238 teams participated in the ICL track. In the second round, 31 teams submitted predictions for the PEFT track, and 17 teams submitted predictions for the ICL track.

4.2 Wining Teams

For both tracks, we rank the teams by the average score of all the 18 sub-tasks in the PromptCBLUE benchmark. In accordance with the regulations of the shared tasks in CHIP-2023, the top-3 teams of each track are eligible for the awards and

---

[5] The PEFT track is at https://tianchi.aliyun.com/competition/entrance/532132, and the ICL track is held at https://tianchi.aliyun.com/competition/entrance/532131.

Table 2. The winning teams and their test results of the PromptCBLUE shared task.

Team name	Rank	Institution	Avg Score
Winners of the PEFT track			
pt.boys	1	Huimei Healthcare Management Services (惠每科技)	71.38
练习一下	2	苏州大学(University of Suzhou) & 北京邮电大学(Beijing University of Posts and Telecommunications)	68.09
Winners of the ICL track			
紫丁香队	1	哈尔滨工业大学(Harbin Institute of Technology)	40.27
ECNU-LLM	2	华东师范大学(East China Normal University)	39.24
IMI1214	3	上海理工大学(University of Shanghai for Science and Technology) & 南京大学(Nanjing University)	36.80

certificates issued by the CHIP-2023 committee. And these teams are invited to submit papers to share their techniques and experiences to the community.[6]

In the Table 2 below, we have listed the top-3 teams from each track. We can see that there is a clear gap between the two tracks with respect to the average score, showing that the open-sourced LLMs can not perform as well as fine-tuning under the ICL setting.

4.3   Methods of the PEFT Track

In this subsection, we will analyze the methods adopted by the top ranked teams in the PEFT track.

Pre-trained Backbones. In this shared task, to ensure fair comparisons and not to turn the whole task to a search of stronger LLM backbone, we only allow the following open-sourced Chinese LLM backbone models: (a) ChatGLM-6B-2[7]; (2) Baichuan-13B-Chat[8]; (3) Chinese-LlaMA2-7B-chat[9]; (4) Chinese-LlaMA2-13B-chat[10]. From the results of the winning teams in the PEFT track, we can

---

[6] The third place of the PEFT track is kept empty since the corresponding team does not submit their materials for review.

[7] https://huggingface.co/THUDM/chatglm2-6b.

[8] https://huggingface.co/baichuan-inc/Baichuan-13B-Chat.

[9] https://huggingface.co/michaelwzhu/Chinese-LlaMA2-chat-7B-sft-v0.3.

[10] https://huggingface.co/michaelwzhu/Chinese-LlaMA2-13B-chat.

see that: (a) the 13B models perform better 7B models under PEFT tuning; (b) the Baichuan-13B-Chat model obtains the strongest performance.

Data Processing and Augmentation. Note that our PromptCBLUE benchmark comes with a training set, and naturally it would enhance the model performance if we conduct certain data augmentation operations on the training set. The following are the data augmentation operations investigated by the winning teams:

- Note that our PromptCBLUE benchmark comes with a training set containing at most 5k to 6.6k samples for each sub-task. However, some tasks from the original CBLUE benchmark have a large training set. Thus, we can augment the training set with the original CBLUE ones. For example, Team pt.boys augments the training sets of the CHIP-CDEE, CMeEE-V2, CHIP-CDN, CMeIE-V2, IMCS-V2-NER, CHIP-MDCFNPC, CHIP-CTC, CHIP-STS and CMedCausal sub-tasks with the CBLUE data by employing the prompt templates open-sourced by us[11]. They augment each of the above mentioned sub-task's training sample size to 16000. To ensure task samples' balance, they also up-sample the other sub-tasks' sample sizes to 8000.
- The previous literature [7,55,58,71] shows that augmenting training samples by randomly masking the contents of the input sentence can improve the robustness of the trained models. Team pt.boys randomly replace the token in the sentence with the <unk> token, for the sentence classification tasks in PromptCBLUE (IMCS-V2-DAC, CHIP-CTC, CHIP-STS, KUAKE-IR, KUAKE-QIC, KUAKE-QQR, and KUAKE-QTR)

The Parameter-Efficient Fine-Tuning Methods. The PEFT methods rises following the rise of pre-trained language models, especially when the research field made efforts to models with larger scales. There are a variety of PEFT methods in the pre-LLM era. However, since the rise of LLMs, especially the open-sourced LLMs, LoRA becomes the most popular PEFT method. We believe that the popularity of LoRA comes from the following three reasons: (a) LoRA is a reparameterization of the original Transformer weights, thus it can be merged to the model backbone and introduce no additional latency; (b) LoRA has a good theoretical basis: it comes from the idea of intrinsic space, and the fact that fine-tuning a well pretrained model is in essence low-rank. (c) open-source implementations. LoRA is implemented by many open-sourced code repositories like the Huggingface PEFT package[12], thus it is very convenient to use. In the PEFT track, all the winning teams use the LoRA method to fine-tune the LLM backbones.

Training Techniques. In order to fine-tune the model properly, a few issues should be addressed. First, despite the fact that most the LLM backbone is

---

[11] The prompt templates of the PromptCBLUE benchmark are open-sourced at https://github.com/michael-wzhu/PromptCBLUE/blob/main/src/data/templ ates_augment.json.

[12] https://github.com/huggingface/peft.

freezed and we only update the LoRA parameters, the LLMs still requires a large GPU memory, which may be difficult to obtain for academia. Thus, Team "联系一下" employ the QLoRA method [5] to reduce the memory requirements during fine-tuning. QLoRA proposes a novel 4-bit quantization method that proves to have minimum effects for the model fine-tuning. In addition, Flash Attention is also applied to reduce the memory consumption when dealing with long sequences. Second, since we are dealing with a multi-task prompt tuning task, many teams pay attention to balance the sample sizes of the subtasks, so that the fine-tuned LLM will perform properly on each subtask.

4.4   Methods of the ICL Track

In this subsection, we will analyze the winning teams' techniques in the ICL track.

Pre-trained Backbones. From the results of the winning teams in the PEFT track, we can see that: (a) similar to the PEFT track, the 13B models perform better 7B models in ICL; (b) Chinese-LlaMA2-13B-chat helps to achieves the best ICL results, showing that Baichuan-13B-Chat is not dominating in every aspects.

Demonstration Selection. The demonstration selection method is the core of the ICL track. When the LLM is a blackbox and can not be fine-tuned, such as model APIs, ICL capabilities play an important role for unseen or emergent tasks. All three winning teams have used the similarity based demonstration selection. That is, for a test prompt, a sentence embedding model is employed to retrieve the most similar prompts in the training set. When computing a similarity score between the test prompt and training sample, different approaches can be employed: (a) traditional methods like BM25 [41]. (b) semantic representation, which relies on a model to transformer the sequences to hidden vectors. Team "紫丁香队" used both methods, and the other two teams mainly rely on the semantic models. Three teams apply different sentence embedding models. For example, Team ECNU-LLM applied the BGE base model [51] for semantic representations and semantic retrieval. When the similar samples are retrieved, there are many approaches to determine the final demonstration combinations:

- The greedy approach. The retrieved top 3–10 training samples are used as demonstrations.
- Knapsack based demonstration selection. Since we are using the LLMs for inference, we have to consider the maximum length it can handle given our GPU environment. Thus, when we have a pre-defined maximum length, choosing the combination of demonstrations becomes a classic knapsack problem if we consider the similarity score of a demonstration as the value, and the sample's length as the item weight. Team "紫丁香队" has investigated this approach and find that this strategy is better than the greedy method on four of the subtasks.

5   Conclusion

In this article, we review the PromptCBLUE benchmark, the first large-scale Chinese medical prompt tuning benchmark. Then, we given an overview of the PromptCBLUE shared task in the CHIP-2023 conference. The shared task is a huge success, attracting participants from both the industry and academia. Then, we analyze the winning methods of the two tracks. Different techniques are investigated in the shared task to fully uncover the limit of the Chinese LLMs.

Acknowledgements. This work was supported by NSFC grants (No. 61972155 and 62136002) and National Key R&D Program of China (No. 2021YFC3340700), and Shanghai Trusted Industry Internet Software Collaborative Innovation Center.

References

1. Beeksma, M., Verberne, S., van den Bosch, A., Das, E., Hendrickx, I., Groenewoud, S.: Predicting life expectancy with a long short-term memory recurrent neural network using electronic medical records. BMC Med. Inform. Decis. Mak. **19**(1), 1–15 (2019)
2. Chen, W., et al.: A benchmark for automatic medical consultation system: frameworks, tasks and datasets. Bioinformatics **39** (2022). https://api.semanticscholar.org/CorpusID:248239674
3. Cui, G., et al.: Ultrafeedback: Boosting language models with high-quality feedback. arXiv abs/2310.01377 (2023). https://api.semanticscholar.org/CorpusID:263605623
4. Dai, D., et al.: Why can GPT learn in-context? Language models secretly perform gradient descent as meta-optimizers. In: Rogers, A., Boyd-Graber, J., Okazaki, N. (eds.) Findings of the Association for Computational Linguistics: ACL 2023, Toronto, Canada, pp. 4005–4019. Association for Computational Linguistics (2023). https://doi.org/10.18653/v1/2023.findings-acl.247. https://aclanthology.org/2023.findings-acl.247
5. Dettmers, T., Pagnoni, A., Holtzman, A., Zettlemoyer, L.: QLoRA: efficient fine-tuning of quantized LLMs. arXiv e-prints arXiv:2305.14314 (2023)
6. Devlin, J., Chang, M.W., Lee, K., Toutanova, K.: BERT: pre-training of deep bidirectional transformers for language understanding. arXiv preprint arXiv:1810.04805 (2018)
7. Feng, S.Y., et al.: A survey of data augmentation approaches for NLP. In: Findings (2021). https://api.semanticscholar.org/CorpusID:234093015
8. Gu, Y., et al.: Domain-specific language model pretraining for biomedical natural language processing (2020)
9. Guan, T., Zan, H., Zhou, X., Xu, H., Zhang, K.: CMeIE: construction and evaluation of Chinese medical information extraction dataset. In: Natural Language Processing and Chinese Computing (2020). https://api.semanticscholar.org/CorpusID:222210416

10. Guo, Z., Ni, Y., Wang, K., Zhu, W., Xie, G.: Global attention decoder for Chinese spelling error correction. In: Findings of the Association for Computational Linguistics: ACL-IJCNLP 2021, pp. 1419–1428 (2021)
11. Hahn, U., Oleynik, M.: Medical information extraction in the age of deep learning. Yearb. Med. Inform. **29**(01), 208–220 (2020)
12. He, J., Zhou, C., Ma, X., Berg-Kirkpatrick, T., Neubig, G.: Towards a unified view of parameter-efficient transfer learning. arXiv abs/2110.04366 (2021)
13. Houlsby, N., et al.: Parameter-efficient transfer learning for NLP. In: International Conference on Machine Learning, pp. 2790–2799. PMLR (2019)
14. Hughes, M., Li, I., Kotoulas, S., Suzumura, T.: Medical text classification using convolutional neural networks. In: Informatics for Health: Connected Citizen-Led Wellness and Population Health, pp. 246–250. IOS Press (2017)
15. Jie, S., Deng, Z.: Convolutional bypasses are better vision transformer adapters. arXiv abs/2207.07039 (2022)
16. Kim, J., et al.: Ground-truth labels matter: A deeper look into input-label demonstrations. arXiv abs/2205.12685 (2022). https://api.semanticscholar.org/CorpusID:249062718
17. Kopiczko, D.J., Blankevoort, T., Asano, Y.M.: Vera: vector-based random matrix adaptation. arXiv abs/2310.11454 (2023). https://api.semanticscholar.org/CorpusID:264172315
18. Le, T., Bertolini, M., No'e, F., Clevert, D.A.: Parameterized hypercomplex graph neural networks for graph classification. In: International Conference on Artificial Neural Networks (2021)
19. Lester, B., Al-Rfou, R., Constant, N.: The power of scale for parameter-efficient prompt tuning. arXiv preprint arXiv:2104.08691 (2021)
20. Levy, I., Bogin, B., Berant, J.: Diverse demonstrations improve in-context compositional generalization. In: Rogers, A., Boyd-Graber, J., Okazaki, N. (eds.) Proceedings of the 61st Annual Meeting of the Association for Computational Linguistics, Toronto, Canada (Volume 1: Long Papers), pp. 1401–1422. Association for Computational Linguistics (2023). https://doi.org/10.18653/v1/2023.acl-long.78. https://aclanthology.org/2023.acl-long.78
21. Li, X.L., Liang, P.: Prefix-tuning: optimizing continuous prompts for generation. In: Proceedings of the 59th Annual Meeting of the Association for Computational Linguistics and the 11th International Joint Conference on Natural Language Processing (Volume 1: Long Papers) abs/2101.00190 (2021)
22. Li, X., et al.: Unified demonstration retriever for in-context learning. arXiv abs/2305.04320 (2023). https://api.semanticscholar.org/CorpusID:258557751
23. Li, X., Qiu, X.: Finding support examples for in-context learning. In: Bouamor, H., Pino, J., Bali, K. (eds.) Findings of the Association for Computational Linguistics: EMNLP 2023, Singapore, pp. 6219–6235. Association for Computational Linguistics (2023). https://doi.org/10.18653/v1/2023.findings-emnlp.411. https://aclanthology.org/2023.findings-emnlp.411
24. Li, Y., Qian, B., Zhang, X., Liu, H.: Graph neural network-based diagnosis prediction. Big Data **8**(5), 379–390 (2020)
25. Li, Z., et al.: CHIP2022 shared task overview: medical causal entity relationship extraction. In: Tang, B., et al. (eds.) CHIP 2022. CCIS, vol. 1773, pp. 51–56. Springer, Singapore (2023). https://doi.org/10.1007/978-981-99-4826-0_5
26. Lin, C.Y.: ROUGE: a package for automatic evaluation of summaries. In: Text Summarization Branches Out, Barcelona, Spain, pp. 74–81. Association for Computational Linguistics (2004). https://aclanthology.org/W04-1013

27. Liu, W., Tang, J., Qin, J., Xu, L., Li, Z., Liang, X.: MedDG: a large-scale medical consultation dataset for building medical dialogue system. arXiv abs/2010.07497 (2020). https://api.semanticscholar.org/CorpusID:222377844

28. Liu, X., Sun, T., Huang, X., Qiu, X.: Late prompt tuning: a late prompt could be better than many prompts. arXiv abs/2210.11292 (2022)

29. Liu, X., Ji, K., Fu, Y., Du, Z., Yang, Z., Tang, J.: P-tuning v2: prompt tuning can be comparable to fine-tuning universally across scales and tasks. arXiv abs/2110.07602 (2021)

30. Liu, X., et al.: P-tuning: prompt tuning can be comparable to fine-tuning across scales and tasks. In: Annual Meeting of the Association for Computational Linguistics (2022)

31. Liu, Z., et al.: LLM360: towards fully transparent open-source LLMs. arXiv e-prints arXiv:2312.06550 (2023)

32. Luo, X., Ni, Y., Tang, B.: Discussion on the application of text semantic matching technology in the field of Chinese medical text from the perspective of competition. China Digit. Med. **11** (2021)

33. Mahabadi, R.K., Henderson, J., Ruder, S.: Compacter: efficient low-rank hyper-complex adapter layers. In: NeurIPS (2021)

34. Min, S., et al.: Rethinking the role of demonstrations: what makes in-context learning work? arXiv abs/2202.12837 (2022). https://api.semanticscholar.org/CorpusID:247155069

35. Moosavi, N.S., Delfosse, Q., Kersting, K., Gurevych, I.: Adaptable adapters. In: North American Chapter of the Association for Computational Linguistics (2022)

36. Ouyang, L., et al.: Training language models to follow instructions with human feedback. In: Advances in Neural Information Processing Systems, vol. 35, pp. 27730–27744 (2022)

37. Pfeiffer, J., Kamath, A., Rücklé, A., Cho, K., Gurevych, I.: AdapterFusion: non-destructive task composition for transfer learning. In: Proceedings of the 16th Conference of the European Chapter of the Association for Computational Linguistics: Main Volume, pp. 487–503. Association for Computational Linguistics, Online (2021). https://doi.org/10.18653/v1/2021.eacl-main.39. https://aclanthology.org/2021.eacl-main.39

38. Qin, C., Zhang, A., Dagar, A., Ye, W.: In-context learning with iterative demonstration selection. arXiv abs/2310.09881 (2023). https://api.semanticscholar.org/CorpusID:264146526

39. Qin, C., Zhang, A., Zhang, Z., Chen, J., Yasunaga, M., Yang, D.: Is Chat-GPT a general-purpose natural language processing task solver? arXiv e-prints arXiv:2302.06476 (2023)

40. Radford, A., Wu, J., Child, R., Luan, D., Amodei, D., Sutskever, I., et al.: Language models are unsupervised multitask learners. OpenAI Blog **1**(8), 9 (2019)

41. Robertson, S.E., Zaragoza, H.: The probabilistic relevance framework: BM25 and beyond. Found. Trends Inf. Retr. **3**, 333–389 (2009). https://api.semanticscholar.org/CorpusID:207178704

42. Rubin, O., Herzig, J., Berant, J.: Learning to retrieve prompts for in-context learning. arXiv abs/2112.08633 (2021). https://api.semanticscholar.org/CorpusID:245218561

43. Rücklé, A., et al.: Adapterdrop: on the efficiency of adapters in transformers. In: Conference on Empirical Methods in Natural Language Processing (2020)

44. Singhal, K., et al.: Large language models encode clinical knowledge. Nature 1–9 (2023)

45. Sung, Y.L., Cho, J., Bansal, M.: LST: ladder side-tuning for parameter and memory efficient transfer learning. arXiv abs/2206.06522 (2022)

46. Vaswani, A., et al.: Attention is all you need. arXiv abs/1706.03762 (2017)

47. Wang, X., Wei, J., Schuurmans, D., Le, Q., Hsin Chi, E.H., Zhou, D.: Self-consistency improves chain of thought reasoning in language models. arXiv abs/2203.11171 (2022). https://api.semanticscholar.org/CorpusID:247595263

48. Wang, X., et al.: Multi-task entity linking with supervision from a taxonomy. Knowl. Inf. Syst. **65**, 4335–4358 (2023). https://api.semanticscholar.org/CorpusID:258975891

49. Wei, J., et al.: Chain of thought prompting elicits reasoning in large language models. arXiv abs/2201.11903 (2022). https://api.semanticscholar.org/CorpusID:246411621

50. Wu, Z., et al.: IDPG: an instance-dependent prompt generation method. In: North American Chapter of the Association for Computational Linguistics (2022)

51. Xiao, S., Liu, Z., Zhang, P., Muennighoff, N.: C-pack: packaged resources to advance general Chinese embedding (2023)

52. Xiong, Y., Chen, M., Chen, Q., Tang, B.: Overview of the CHIP2021 shared task 1: classifying positive and negative clinical findings in medical dialog. In: China Health Information Processing Conference (2021)

53. Yao, Y., Duan, J., Xu, K., Cai, Y., Sun, E., Zhang, Y.: A survey on large language model (LLM) security and privacy: the good, the bad, and the ugly. arXiv abs/2312.02003 (2023). https://api.semanticscholar.org/CorpusID:265609409

54. Zan, H., Li, W., Zhang, K., Ye, Y., Chang, B., Sui, Z.: Building a pediatric medical corpus: word segmentation and named entity annotation. In: Chinese Lexical Semantics (2020). https://api.semanticscholar.org/CorpusID:236477750

55. Zhang, J., Tan, M., Dai, P., Zhu, W.G.: LECO: improving early exiting via learned exits and comparison-based exiting mechanism. In: Annual Meeting of the Association for Computational Linguistics (2023). https://api.semanticscholar.org/CorpusID:259370796

56. Zhang, L., Zhang, L., Shi, S., Chu, X., Li, B.: LoRA-FA: memory-efficient low-rank adaptation for large language models fine-tuning. arXiv abs/2308.03303 (2023). https://api.semanticscholar.org/CorpusID:260683267

57. Zhang, N., et al.: CBLUE: a Chinese biomedical language understanding evaluation benchmark. In: Proceedings of the 60th Annual Meeting of the Association for Computational Linguistics, Dublin, Ireland (Volume 1: Long Papers), pp. 7888–7915. Association for Computational Linguistics (2022). https://doi.org/10.18653/v1/2022.acl-long.544. https://aclanthology.org/2022.acl-long.544

58. Zhang, X., Tan, M., Zhang, J., Zhu, W.: NAG-NER: a unified non-autoregressive generation framework for various NER tasks. In: Annual Meeting of the Association for Computational Linguistics (2023). https://api.semanticscholar.org/CorpusID:259370837

59. Zhang, Y., Gao, X., Zhu, W., Wang, X.: FastNER: speeding up inferences for named entity recognition tasks. In: International Conference on Advanced Data Mining and Applications (2023). https://api.semanticscholar.org/CorpusID:265214231

60. Zhang, Y., Wang, P., Tan, M., Zhu, W.G.: Learned adapters are better than manually designed adapters. In: Annual Meeting of the Association for Computational Linguistics (2023). https://api.semanticscholar.org/CorpusID:259858833

61. Zhang, Z., Zhu, W., Yan, J., Gao, P., Xie, G.: Automatic student network search for knowledge distillation. In: 2020 25th International Conference on Pattern Recognition (ICPR), pp. 2446–2453 (2021)

62. Zhao, W.X., et al.: A survey of large language models. arXiv e-prints arXiv:2303.18223 (2023)

63. Zheng, H., Zhu, W., Wang, P., Wang, X.: Candidate soups: fusing candidate results improves translation quality for non-autoregressive translation. arXiv abs/2301.11503 (2023). https://api.semanticscholar.org/CorpusID:256358677

64. Zhou, B., Yang, G., Shi, Z., Ma, S.: Natural language processing for smart healthcare. arXiv e-prints arXiv:2110.15803 (2021)

65. Zhou, X., et al.: Analysis of the health information needs of diabetics in China. Stud. Health Technol. Inform. **264**, 487–491 (2019). https://api.semanticscholar.org/CorpusID:201617388

66. Zhu, W.: AutoNLU: architecture search for sentence and cross-sentence attention modeling with re-designed search space. In: Natural Language Processing and Chinese Computing (2021). https://api.semanticscholar.org/CorpusID:238862030

67. Zhu, W.: MVP-BERT: multi-vocab pre-training for Chinese BERT. In: Proceedings of the 59th Annual Meeting of the Association for Computational Linguistics and the 11th International Joint Conference on Natural Language Processing: Student Research Workshop, pp. 260–269. Association for Computational Linguistics, Online (2021). https://doi.org/10.18653/v1/2021.acl-srw.27. https://aclanthology.org/2021.acl-srw.27

68. Zhu, W.: MVP-BERT: multi-vocab pre-training for Chinese BERT. In: Annual Meeting of the Association for Computational Linguistics (2021). https://api.semanticscholar.org/CorpusID:237331564

69. Zhu, W., et al.: paht_nlp @ mediqa 2021: multi-grained query focused multi-answer summarization. In: Workshop on Biomedical Natural Language Processing (2021). https://api.semanticscholar.org/CorpusID:235097590

70. Zhu, W., et al.: Extracting decision trees from medical texts: An overview of the text2dt track in CHIP2022. In: Tang, B., et al. (eds.) CHIP 2022. CCIS, vol. 1773, pp. 89–102. Springer, Singapore (2023). https://doi.org/10.1007/978-981-99-4826-0_9

71. Zhu, W., Ni, Y., Wang, X., Xie, G.: Discovering better model architectures for medical query understanding. In: Proceedings of the 2021 Conference of the North American Chapter of the Association for Computational Linguistics: Human Language Technologies: Industry Papers, pp. 230–237. Association for Computational Linguistics, Online (2021). https://doi.org/10.18653/v1/2021.naacl-industry.29. https://aclanthology.org/2021.naacl-industry.29

72. Zhu, W., Tan, M.: SPT: learning to selectively insert prompts for better prompt tuning. In: Bouamor, H., Pino, J., Bali, K. (eds.) Proceedings of the 2023 Conference on Empirical Methods in Natural Language Processing, Singapore, pp. 11862–11878. Association for Computational Linguistics (2023). https://aclanthology.org/2023.emnlp-main.727

73. Zhu, W., Wang, P., Ni, Y., Xie, G.T., Wang, X.: Badge: speeding up BERT inference after deployment via block-wise bypasses and divergence-based early exiting. In: Annual Meeting of the Association for Computational Linguistics (2023). https://api.semanticscholar.org/CorpusID:259370582

74. Zhu, W., Wang, X.: ChatMed: a Chinese medical large language model (2023). https://github.com/michael-wzhu/ChatMed

75. Zhu, W., Wang, X., Ni, Y., Xie, G.: AutoTrans: automating transformer design via reinforced architecture search. In: Wang, L., Feng, Y., Hong, Yu., He, R. (eds.) NLPCC 2021. LNCS (LNAI), vol. 13028, pp. 169–182. Springer, Cham (2021). https://doi.org/10.1007/978-3-030-88480-2_14

76. Zhu, W., Wang, X., Zheng, H., Chen, M., Tang, B.: PromptCBLUE: a Chinese prompt tuning benchmark for the medical domain. arXiv e-prints arXiv:2310.14151 (2023)
77. Zong, H., Yang, J., Zhang, Z., Li, Z., Zhang, X.: Semantic categorization of Chinese eligibility criteria in clinical trials using machine learning methods. BMC Med. Inform. Decis. Making **21** (2021). https://api.semanticscholar.org/CorpusID: 233239370

Innovative Design of Large Language Model in the Medical Field Based on chip-PromptCBLUE

Hongshun Ling, Bin Yin, Chengze Ge, PengTao Shi, Jie Wang, Xian Fan, and Fuliang Quan[✉]

Huimei Technology, Hangzhou, China
{linghongshun,yinbin,gechengze,quanfuliang}@huimei.com

Abstract. This article introduces the research content and results based on the CHIP-PromptCBLUE (Chinese Biomedical Language Understanding Evaluation) benchmark task. PromptCBLUE promotes research on large language models for medicine. The benchmark can evaluate Chinese language models' multi-tasking abilities across various medical tasks, including 18 task types such as medical entity recognition, medical text classification, medical language inference, and medical content generation. It requires completing all tasks using just one large language model, necessitating efficient fine-tuning methods and keeping parameters within 1% of the model size. To address this, we propose a method. First, we greatly improved model performance through data augmentation. We then further amplified model capabilities using an innovative entity loss optimization of the large model's loss function. Using this method, we achieved a score of 71.3822 in the chip-PromptCBLUE general track. This research provides new ideas for advancing large language models in the medical field.

Keywords: LLM · chip-promptCBLUE · PEFT

1 Introduction

CHIP-PromptCBLUE [14] benchmark is an upgraded version of CBLUE (Chinese Biomedical Language Understanding Evaluation), consisting of 18 subtasks across 4 major categories: medical entity recognition, medical text classification, medical language inference, and medical content generation. Compared to CCKS-PromptCBLUE's [15] LLM evaluation tasks, PromptCBLUE has been fully upgraded. PromptCBLUE adds two challenging CBLUE tasks: Text2DT and CMedCausal. These two tasks require in-depth understanding of medical texts and have complex output forms, posing challenges for LLMs. The prompt templates involved in CCKS-PromptCBLUE test set only have 94 templates, while CHIP-PromptCBLUE will have 450 templates, imposing higher robustness requirements on LLMs. Efficient fine-tuning modules need to be added on

---

H. Ling and B. Yin—Contributed equally to this work.

H. Xu et al. (Eds.): CHIP 2023, CCIS 2080, pp. 21–30, 2024.
https://doi.org/10.1007/978-981-97-1717-0_2

top of the open-sourced major model backbone, with the additional parameters no more than 1% of the major model parameters. Only the efficient fine-tuning modules can be fine-tuned without modifying the major model backbone. And only one set of efficient fine-tuning modules can be used to complete all tasks, thus imposing higher requirements on the large language models.

Large language models have powerful understanding and generation capabilities in the medical field. Through pre-training, they gain profound understanding of natural language and can better analyze complex medical texts and generate high-quality responses. Large language models can learn comprehensive medical knowledge graphs through massive corpora and have strong medical logical reasoning abilities. First, we significantly improved the overall model performance by using data augmentation on 8 tasks including CHIP-CDEE, CMeEE-V2, CHIP-CDN, CMeIE-V2, IMCS-V2-NER, CHIP-MDCFNPC, CHIP-CTC, CHIP-STS, CMedCausal. Also, for tasks like CMeIE-V2, CHIP-CDEE, CMeEE-V2 that have fixed extraction patterns, we innovatively optimized the loss function, further enhancing model performance. The application of large language models in medicine provides new ideas for the development of this field.

2   Related Work

In recent years, the pre-training and fine-tuning framework has become the standard paradigm for natural language processing (NLP) tasks. BERT [3] conducts large-scale unsupervised pre-training using masked language modeling to learn language representations. T5 [10] converts various NLP tasks into text-to-text format, demonstrating multi-task learning abilities. GPT-3 [1] utilizes huge transformer models for autoregressive prediction and introduces prompt-based learning. These models prove the effectiveness of pre-training and fine-tuning, and have achieved better performance with increasing model size. The pre-training and fine-tuning framework is widely applied in NLP and can be extended to computer vision and other domains, providing new possibilities for language understanding in professional fields like healthcare.

In the new wave of AI development, large models have been applied across various fields and industries. OpenAI proposed InstructGPT [9], a system built on large language models (LLMs), which utilizes human feedback for fine-tuning and reinforcement learning to generate outputs that better conform to human expectations and are more realistic. The InstructGPT training process includes supervised fine-tuning and reinforcement learning stages. In supervised fine-tuning, the model is fine-tuned using human annotated instruction-response examples. The reinforcement learning stage constructs a reward model to evaluate the quality of generated responses. Human annotators rank preferences over different responses to the same input, and the reward model is trained on these rankings. In reinforcement learning, the reward model acts as the reward function and proximal policy optimization (PPO) is used for training. Meanwhile, a penalty on the KL divergence from the original fine-tuned model is applied to prevent the model from deviating from the original semantic space.

With human feedback fine-tuning and reinforcement learning, InstructGPT generates responses that better conform to instructions, are more realistic, and exhibit improved persona consistency in multi-turn interactions. The Instruct-GPT research shows that leveraging human feedback is an effective way to improve large language models in following interactive instructions, generating realism, and ensuring safety. This provides valuable experience and inspiration for language generation tasks in healthcare. Experiments on the Text2MDT [13] task are conducted using prompting methods for large language models, and a pipeline framework that decomposes the task into three subtasks is proposed. UDR [6] proposes a unified demonstration retriever applied to large language models which improves performance.

LoRA (Low-Rank Adaptation) [4] is an efficient fine-tuning method for large-scale language models. Usually, fine-tuning large models requires extensive compute resources. LoRA introduces low-rank adaptation modules after each transformer block for adaptation. The parameters in the adaptation modules are much smaller than the original model. Only the adaptation module parameters are fine-tuned rather than the whole model. The LoRA adaptation matrix is decomposed into the product of two low-rank matrices using low-rank decomposition. This reduces the parameters and computations in the adaptation modules. LoRA only updates the low-rank parameters in the adaptation modules, allowing fine-tuning large models within smaller GPU memory and with higher efficiency. Experiments show that compared to direct full model fine-tuning, LoRA reduces fine-tuned parameters by over 75% and computations by over 80%, while achieving comparable performance. The LoRA research demonstrates that for large language model fine-tuning, the ideas of low-rank decomposition and modular adaptation can significantly reduce the compute and memory requirements, enabling more efficient large model fine-tuning. This parameter-efficient fine-tuning approach provides an important path to deploy large models under resource constraints. Other Parameter-Efficient Fine-Tuning Methods such as qlora [2], P-Tuning [8], P-Tuning v2 [7], Prefix-Tuning [5] and BitFit [12] optimize different target structures of large models for efficient fine-tuning.

3   Method

Our method is based on efficient fine-tuning with LoRA, where the LoRA adaptation modules use low-rank decomposition to factorize the adaptation matrix into the product of two low-rank matrices. This reduces the parameters for fine-tuning and achieves comparable performance to full-parameter fine-tuning of the base model, providing high cost-effectiveness.

Prompts need to be constructed as model input before large model predictions. Good prompts can significantly improve the quality of model generations and output responses that better meet user needs, enabling better human-machine interaction. Constructing high-quality prompts requires clearly stating the task objective, expressing the specific task for the model concisely and unambiguously; using natural language with clear, complete statements rather than keywords, and a friendly tone without commands; controlling length to around 50 words typically to avoid overloading information. The SELF-INSTRUCT [11] framework can help improve model performance by utilizing the model's own generated instructions to increase diversity.

Firstly, for this evaluation task, data augmentation was used to improve model performance. Increasing the sample amount and diversity enhances the model's ability to extract contexts and generalize, serving as an important means to improve model effectiveness. Secondly, for tasks with specific patterns like entity extraction and relation identification, introducing keyword loss in the model's loss function can guide the model to learn and memorize key information more focusedly, thus improving downstream task performance. Meanwhile, the proportion of keyword loss needs to be properly controlled to avoid overfitting on certain keywords.

3.1 Prompt Construction

The organizer provided prompts for different tasks in CHIP-PromptCBLUE. These instructions guide the large model to perform corresponding task identification and generate results for that task. Take the named entity recognition task in CMeEE-V2 as an example for prompt construction, as shown in the figure. To adapt the task for the instructional input and text-form answers of large models, some modifications were made. The original CMeEE-V2 sample has the natural language electronic medical record as input, and output in JSON format, defining the position start and end, entity type and entity name for named entities.

The CMeEE-V2 task prompt is "Find the specified entity: [INPUT-TEXT] Type options: [NER-TYPE] Answer:". This prompt has two slots INPUT-TEXT and NER-TYPE that can be filled in. INPUT-TEXT is filled with the input electronic medical record, and NER-TYPE is replaced by candidate named entity types.

For the output template "The entities contained in the above sentence include: [NER1-TYPE]: [NER1-LIST] [NER2-TYPE]: [NER2-LIST]", based on the JSON output format, named entities can be aggregated by type, then NER1-TYPE is replaced by the entity type, and NER1-LIST filled with the list of entity names for that type.

Through such modifications, the task can be adapted for the instructional input and text-form answers of large models.

3.2 Data Amplification

The training data categories of chip-promptCblue consist of 4 major categories and 18 subtasks, including medical entity recognition, medical text classification, medical language inference and medical content generation, with a total of 82,600 data samples, averaging around 4,500 samples per task. From the public CBLUE datasets, we observed that some tasks have much more data than the evaluation tasks, and there is duplication of the same medical sample reused across different evaluation tasks by constructing new training samples with different prompts. Therefore, data amplification can be used to expand the data and achieve diversity in the training samples, enhancing the model's ability to extract contexts and generalize. We significantly improved the overall model performance by using data amplification techniques on 8 tasks including CHIP-CDEE, CMeEE-V2, CHIP-CDN, CMeIE-V2, IMCS-V2-NER, CHIP-MDCFNPC, CHIP-CTC, CHIP-STS, CMedCausal.

As shown in Fig. 1, the data amplification is divided into five steps. First, prompt templates are obtained for the 8 tasks. Second, instructions for the large model are constructed following the method introduced in Sect. 3.1 Prompt Construction. Third, 16,000 samples are randomly sampled for the data amplification tasks, while 8,000 samples are randomly sampled for the tasks without data amplification. Finally, the sampled results from both parts are used as training data.

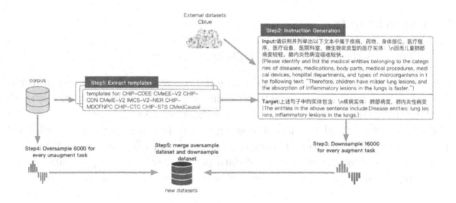

Fig. 1. Data amplification steps

3.3   Entity Loss

The baseline loss is only based on token-level cross-entropy, while the improvement is to introduce loss on entity and entity type positions, in order to make the model pay more attention to key entity and entity type information.

For example, for the following case label: "Entities in the above sentence: Disease entities: GBS cellulitis, lymphadenitis Bodily site entities: face, mandible, inguinal area, scrotum, pubic bone", the key information is the entities 'Disease', 'GBS cellulitis', 'lymphadenitis', 'Bodily site', 'face', 'mandible', 'inguinal area', 'scrotum', 'pubic bone' and the entity type information.

The vector c is used to represent the token loss component. Since cross-entropy loss requires computation for each token position, c is a constant vector with all elements set to 1.

$$c = \begin{bmatrix} 1 & 1 & \cdots & 1 \end{bmatrix} \tag{1}$$

The vector **mask** represents the tokens that need to be considered for entity loss. Each element m_i can take on the values 0 or 1, where 0 indicates an unimportant token and 1 indicates an important token.

$$mask = \begin{bmatrix} m_0 & m_1 & \cdots & m_n \end{bmatrix} \qquad (2)$$

Finally, the vector **mask** is added element-wise to the vector **c** and multiplied by the cross-entropy loss, and λ is a constant parameter used to represent the proportion of the entity loss when adding two losses. A larger λ indicates a higher weight of the entity loss, and vice versa. Here, i represents each token position, len is the number of tokens, a is the word index in the dictionary, and M is the size of the dictionary. The total loss is represented by the following equation:

$$(\lambda \cdot mask + c) \times \sum_{i}^{len} \sum_{c=1}^{M} y_{ia} log(P_{ia}) \qquad (3)$$

4   Experiments

4.1   Datasets and Evaluation Metrics

The dataset consists of 18 subtasks across major categories of medical information extraction (entity recognition, relation extraction, event extraction), medical term normalization, medical text classification, medical sentence semantic relation judgment, and medical dialog understanding and generation. Figure 2 shows the data distribution across tasks before and after augmentation. The inner circles represent the amount of data per task prior to augmentation. The outer rings depict the increased data volume per task following augmentation.

4.2   Experimental Setup

On chip-promptCBLUE, we used baichuan-13b-chat as the large language model backbone and LoRA for efficient fine-tuning. The LoRA parameters were set as

$$lora\_target = \text{`}W\_pack, o\_proj, gate\_proj, up\_proj, down\_proj\text{'}$$
$$lora\_rank = 8, lora\_alpha : 32, lora\_dropout : 0.1.$$

Other training parameters were: number of epochs=5, λ for entity loss=0.25, lr_scheduler='cosine'. Finally, the trainable params for LoRA were 27893760, all params for the large language model were 13292794880, and the trainable params ratio was 0.2098%, which is less than the competition requirement of 1%.

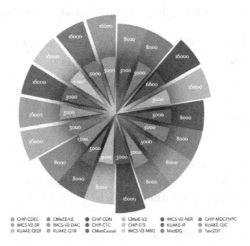

Fig. 2. Data distribution

4.3 Results

In the baseline, only LoRA was used for supervised fine-tuning, achieving an average score of 0.6525 across the 18 tasks. First, supervised fine-tuning with data augmentation was used, improving the average score to 0.7001 (+0.0232). Finally, incorporating the entity_loss, the average score reached 0.7138 (+0.0082). Overall performance are presented in Table 1.

Table 1. Overall Performance

Method	performance (%)
only lora supervised fine-tuning(baseline)	65.25
data amplification(ours)	70.01
entity_loss+data amplification(ours)	**71.38**

4.4 Ablation Study

We conducted ablation studies on two aspects for the data augmentation task: the amount of augmented data and the lambda parameter for the entity loss.

Data Amplification. For the amount of augmented data, the experiments in Table 2 showed that too little data amplification results in insufficient diversity of the training samples and insignificant performance improvement. On the other hand, too much augmentation generates a lot of redundant data for training. The diversity does not improve but is like training for more epochs, which can easily lead to overfitting and decreased test set performance.

Table 2. Ablation Experiments on Data Amplification

Data Amplification Quantity	performance (%)
8,000	66.14
12,000	68.38
16,000	**70.01**
20,000	69.27

Entity Loss. There is a lambda parameter in the entity_loss to adjust the proportion of entity_loss in the total_loss. The larger the lambda, the more the model focuses on key entity information.

Table 3. Ablation Experiments on Entity Loss

the Parameter of Lambda	performance (%)
0	70.01
0.1	70.53
0.25	**71.38**
0.5	70.82
1.0	69.57

The experiments in Table 3 show that a lambda value of 0.25 works best. Although larger lambda values make the model pay more attention to key entities, it can lead to incorrect syntactic generation, causing the post-processing code to fail to parse entities.

5   Conclusion

This article presents a method for optimizing large language models for the chip-PromptCBLUE evaluation task. Firstly, by augmenting data in eight tasks including CHIP-CDEE, CMeEE-V2, CHIP-CDN, CMeIE-V2, IMCS-V2-NER, the scores were improved to 0.7001. Finally, by integrating the entity loss mechanism into the model's loss calculation, the score was further increased to 0.7138. This work explores unique and innovative approaches in the design of large-scale language model applications in the medical field.

References

1. Brown, T.B., et al.: Language models are few-shot learners. In: Larochelle, H., Ranzato, M., Hadsell, R., Balcan, M., Lin, H. (eds.) Advances in Neural Information Processing Systems 33: Annual Conference on Neural Information Processing Systems 2020, NeurIPS 2020, pp. 6–12, 2020. Virtual (2020). https://proceedings.neurips.cc/paper/2020/hash/1457c0d6bfcb4967418bfb8ac142f64a-Abstract.html

2. Dettmers, T., Pagnoni, A., Holtzman, A., Zettlemoyer, L.: QLORA: efficient finetuning of quantized LLMs. CoRR abs/2305.14314 (2023). https://doi.org/10.48550/ARXIV.2305.14314

3. Devlin, J., Chang, M., Lee, K., Toutanova, K.: BERT: pre-training of deep bidirectional transformers for language understanding. In: Burstein, J., Doran, C., Solorio, T. (eds.) Proceedings of the 2019 Conference of the North American Chapter of the Association for Computational Linguistics: Human Language Technologies, NAACL-HLT 2019, Minneapolis, MN, USA, 2–7 June 2019 (Volume 1: Long and Short Papers), pp. 4171–4186. Association for Computational Linguistics (2019). https://doi.org/10.18653/V1/N19-1423

4. Hu, E.J., et al.: LoRA: low-rank adaptation of large language models. In: The Tenth International Conference on Learning Representations, ICLR 2022, Virtual Event, 25–29 April 2022. OpenReview.net (2022). https://openreview.net/forum?id=nZeVKeeFYf9

5. Li, X.L., Liang, P.: Prefix-tuning: optimizing continuous prompts for generation. In: Zong, C., Xia, F., Li, W., Navigli, R. (eds.) Proceedings of the 59th Annual Meeting of the Association for Computational Linguistics and the 11th International Joint Conference on Natural Language Processing, ACL/IJCNLP 2021 (Volume 1: Long Papers), Virtual Event, 1–6 August 2021, pp. 4582–4597. Association for Computational Linguistics (2021). https://doi.org/10.18653/V1/2021.ACL-LONG.353

6. Li, X., et al.: Unified demonstration retriever for in-context learning. In: Rogers, A., Boyd-Graber, J.L., Okazaki, N. (eds.) Proceedings of the 61st Annual Meeting of the Association for Computational Linguistics (Volume 1: Long Papers), ACL 2023, Toronto, Canada, 9–14 July 2023, pp. 4644–4668. Association for Computational Linguistics (2023). https://doi.org/10.18653/V1/2023.ACL-LONG.256

7. Liu, X., Ji, K., Fu, Y., Du, Z., Yang, Z., Tang, J.: P-tuning v2: prompt tuning can be comparable to fine-tuning universally across scales and tasks. CoRR abs/2110.07602 (2021). https://arxiv.org/abs/2110.07602

8. Liu, X., et al.: P-tuning: prompt tuning can be comparable to fine-tuning across scales and tasks. In: Muresan, S., Nakov, P., Villavicencio, A. (eds.) Proceedings of the 60th Annual Meeting of the Association for Computational Linguistics (Volume 2: Short Papers), ACL 2022, Dublin, Ireland, 22–27 May 2022, pp. 61–68. Association for Computational Linguistics (2022). https://doi.org/10.18653/V1/2022.ACL-SHORT.8

9. Ouyang, L., et al.: Training language models to follow instructions with human feedback. In: NeurIPS (2022). http://papers.nips.cc/paper_files/paper/2022/hash/b1efde53be364a73914f58805a001731-Abstract-Conference.html

10. Raffel, C., et al.: Exploring the limits of transfer learning with a unified text-to-text transformer. J. Mach. Learn. Res. **21**, 140:1–140:67 (2020). http://jmlr.org/papers/v21/20-074.html

11. Wang, Y., et al.: Self-instruct: aligning language models with self-generated instructions. In: Rogers, A., Boyd-Graber, J.L., Okazaki, N. (eds.) Proceedings of the 61st Annual Meeting of the Association for Computational Linguistics (Volume 1: Long Papers), ACL 2023, Toronto, Canada, 9–14 July 2023, pp. 13484–13508. Association for Computational Linguistics (2023). https://doi.org/10.18653/V1/2023.ACL-LONG.754

12. Zaken, E.B., Goldberg, Y., Ravfogel, S.: BitFit: simple parameter-efficient finetuning for transformer-based masked language-models. In: Muresan, S., Nakov, P., Villavicencio, A. (eds.) Proceedings of the 60th Annual Meeting of the Association for Computational Linguistics (Volume 2: Short Papers), ACL 2022, Dublin, Ire-

land, 22–27 May 2022, pp. 1–9. Association for Computational Linguistics (2022). https://doi.org/10.18653/V1/2022.ACL-SHORT.1

13. Zhu, W., et al.: Text2MDT: extracting medical decision trees from medical texts (2024)

14. Zhu, W., Wang, X., Chen, M., Tang, B.: Overview of the promptCBLUE shared task in CHIP2023 (2023)

15. Zhu, W., Wang, X., Zheng, H., Chen, M., Tang, B.: PromptCBLUE: a Chinese prompt tuning benchmark for the medical domain (2023)

CMed-Baichuan: Task Explanation-Enhanced Prompt Method on PromptCBLUE Benchmark

Xinyuan Ren[1,2], Yilin Song[3], Chenwei Yan[1,2(✉)], Yuxuan Xiong[1,2],
Fang Kong[3(✉)], and Xiangling Fu[1,2]

[1] School of Computer Science (National Pilot Software Engineering School),
Beijing University of Posts and Telecommunications, Beijing, China
[2] Key Laboratory of Trustworthy Distributed Computing and Service (BUPT),
Ministry of Education, Beijing, China
{chenwei.yan,bupt_xyx,fuxiangling}@bupt.edu.cn
[3] School of Computer Science, Soochow University, Suzhou, China
kongfang@suda.edu.cn

Abstract. Large Language Models (LLMs) have received widespread attention from academia and industry for their excellent performance on NLP tasks. Due to the knowledge-intensive nature of the medical field, previous studies proposed various fine-tuning methods and fine-tuned domain LLMs to align the general LLMs into specific domains. However, they ignored the difficulty of understanding the medical task requirements, that is LLMs are expected to give answers in the situation of not fully understanding the requirements of the task itself and instructions. So, in this paper, we argue that the explanation of task requirements is important to improve LLM's understanding. Moreover, we proposed a task explanation-enhanced prompt method and introduced a medical LLM, CMed-Baichuan. In addition, we evaluated our model on the PromptCBLUE benchmark, which is the first LLM evaluation benchmark covering 18 Chinese medical NLP tasks, and the experimental results show that our model achieved state-of-the-art performance on overall score, and also demonstrate the importance of task explanation. Our code is publicly available at https://github.com/naginoa/CMed-Baichuan.

Keywords: Large Language Models · LLM Evaluation · Medical LLM · Prompt

1 Introduction

Recently, large language models (LLMs) represented by chatGPT[1] have received widespread attention from academia and industry. With the evolution of the

---

[1] https://chat.openai.com.chat.

X. Ren and Y. Song—These authors contributed equally to this work.

© The Author(s), under exclusive license to Springer Nature Singapore Pte Ltd. 2024
H. Xu et al. (Eds.): CHIP 2023, CCIS 2080, pp. 31–48, 2024.
https://doi.org/10.1007/978-981-97-1717-0_3

GPT-3 [2] and its successors, such as PaLM [4], OPT [34], LLaMA [23] and GPT-4 [16], LLMs demonstrated impressive performance across various tasks, for example, machine translation [38] and question answering [10]. Previous studies show that LLMs can absorb experience and knowledge from a massive unlabelled corpus and have emergent abilities [28], thus many traditional methods in natural language processing (NLP) are challenged by LLM-based methods.

To align the general LLMs into specific domains, many fine-tuning methods are applied. In the medical domain, Singhal et al. [21] proposed instruction prompt tuning and introduced the resulting model Med-PaLM. Hongbo et al. [32] proposed HuaTuoGPT, which is based on LLaMa-7B and integrates medical knowledge from the Chinese Medical Knowledge Graph (CMeKG) for fine-tuning. The results prove that the models fine-tuned on specific domain data often outperform the general ones, but there is still a gap with human levels. These methods are effective and demonstrate the importance of knowledge as well. That is, since the medical domain is such a knowledge-intensive domain, the barriers to entry in the medical field are high, and many tasks require higher understanding and specific domain knowledge.

However, for medical domains, the explanation of the task is also important to help LLMs improve their understanding, which is ignored by many current methods. In particular, many medical tasks are complex, and current emergent capabilities in LLMs may not support their full understanding of the requirements of the task itself and instructions. In that case, it is difficult for LLMs to provide satisfactory answers.

Moreover, in the medical domain, existing evaluation studies focus more on a few tasks [21], such as medical exams and medical online question answering, many typical medical tasks are not covered. A more comprehensive evaluation of different medical tasks is needed to understand the capabilities and limitations of large language models.

Thus, in this paper, to gain a better understanding of the capabilities of LLMs for medical tasks, and improve the performance of medical LLMs as well, we conduct an evaluation of various medical tasks and propose a task explanation-enhanced prompt method to fine-tune general LLM. The main contribution can be summarized below.

- We provide an overview of medical benchmark, PromptCBLUE in the form of a unified task, which transformed 18 medical NLP tasks into prompt-based language generation tasks, and evaluate three typical open-source LLMs on it.
- We propose a task explanation-enhanced prompt method to improve the understanding ability of LLMs on specific domains, which is vital to knowledge-intensive domains.
- We introduce a fine-tuned medical LLM, CMed-Baichuan, to adapt the LLM to medical tasks. The experimental results show that our fine-tuned LLM achieves state-of-art performance on the average score on 18 tasks, where achieves the best performance in 13 tasks, and competitive performance on the rest 5 tasks.

2 Related Work

2.1 Large Language Models

Recently, the emerging large language models (LLMs) [2,16,17,23] have received widespread attention from academia and industry. They are trained on large-scale data by in-context learning to optimize massive billion-level parameter and provides a powerful tool for natural language understanding and generation tasks. GPT-3 used 175 billion parameters (175B) [7], while the parameter sizes of PaLM [4] and GPT-4 [16] reach 540 billion and 1.76 trillion, respectively. Besides, the widely-used open-source LLMs include LLaMA (7B to 70B [23,24]), GLM (6B to 130B [6,31]), Baichuan (7B to 13B [1]) and etc.

Some studies have proved that LLMs show emergent abilities with the model scale increased [18,28], and many LLMs show impressive performance on real-world tasks. Therefore, there is a growing trend of shifting traditional NLP tasks towards generative tasks, wherein LLMs are tasked with providing answers directly. As for how to transform the traditional NLP tasks to the input and output format of LLMs, the methods are various. For the natural language generation tasks, such as text summarization and translation tasks, there are nearly no additional changes except for a prompt to instruct the model to produce the corresponding output. This transformation also applies to reading comprehension tasks and question answering tasks. For text classification tasks, all labels should be given in the prompt. However, it is not easy to transform the information retrieval tasks to adapt to LLMs due to the massive candidate text [30]. Further, the traditional input and output formats are both changed in information extraction tasks. For example, LLMs are required to give named entities mentioned in text and results are often insufficient which ignores the location and BIO tagging scheme. In summary, some tasks are naturally adapted to large models, but others require task transformation and inappropriate transformation may not fully stimulate the capacities and potential of LLMs.

2.2 Tuning on Large Language Models

LLMs can be better adapted to specific tasks by exploiting different tuning techniques. Prompt tuning is a simple and intuitive mechanism. At first, hard prompts are used to interact with LLMs with frozen parameters, which generates task-oriented static templates [2,20,22,29]. Subsequently, many studies [15,19] introduce soft prompts, which exploit continuous trainable vectors to replace discrete input tokens. Li and Liang [13] proposed the prefix-tuning method which optimizes a continuous task-specific vector with LLM parameters frozen. Lester et al. [11] demonstrate the effectiveness of prompt ensembling. Moreover, Wei et al. [27] proposed instruction tuning to improve zero-shot learning. Singhal et al. proposed [21] instruction prompt-tuning to align general LLM to the medical domain with a small amount of data. Hu et al. [9] introduced Low-Rank Adaptation (LoRA) to reduce the trainable parameters by rank decomposition matrices.

2.3 Evaluation on LLMs

With the development of LLMs and their applications, such as summarization, translation, and sentiment analysis [8,38], there is an increasing need to evaluate existing LLMs on various benchmarks. Thus, some studies have emerged to evaluate the LLMs from the aspects of understanding, reasoning, coherence, robustness, trustworthiness, hallucinations, ethics, etc. [3,14,21,26].

From the perspective of evaluation methods, the evaluation can be categorized as human-based methods, signal-based methods, and automatic evaluation [12,26]. From the perspective of evaluation objects, some are for general domain, while others are limited to specific domains. In the medical domain, most studies are limited to a small number of medical tasks. Singhal et al. [21] evaluated several medical question answering benchmarks, but other classic medical tasks are not covered. In addition, due to the difficulty in the disclosure and labeling of medical data, it is hard to conduct a comprehensive study.

3 PromptCBLUE Benchmark and Metrics

3.1 Benchmark Description

With the popularity of LLMs, almost all NLP tasks have been transformed into prompt-based language generation tasks. PromptCBLUE[2] [36,37], a secondary development dataset of the CBLUE benchmark [33], provides an evaluation benchmark in the form of a unified Chinese medical NLP task.

It converts 18 different medical NLP tasks into prompt-based language generation tasks, forming the first LLM evaluation benchmark for Chinese medical NLP tasks. The overview of this benchmark and detailed description are summarized in Table 1.

3.2 Task Transformation

To make it clear, we summarize these 18 tasks into six categories: Information Extraction, Classification, Semantic Matching, Text Generation, Tree Generation, and Complex Tasks. The detailed description of each task is shown in Table 1. Next, we will introduce how these tasks are transformed into a new format to adapt to the input and output requirements of LLMs.

Information Extraction. For information extraction tasks, the form of sequences is no longer used, but more explicit information is given in the input. Specifically, LLMs are required to generate entity mention based on the specified entity type, and the position of the span is not needed in the NER task, while the relationship type should be given in the triple extraction task.

Classification. For classification tasks, it is treated as a multi-choice question and the labels are regarded as candidate options. For intent detection tasks, the

---

[2] https://github.com/michael-wzhu/PromptCBLUE.

Table 1. The detailed description of the PromptCBLUE benchmark and the metrics for each task. The main metrics of each task are highlighted in **bold**.

Index	Category	Dataset	Task Type&Description	Metrics
1	Information	CMeEE	NER	Micro Precision,
2	Extraction	IMCS-NER	NER	Micro Recall,
3		CMeIE	Triple extraction	**Micro F1 Scores**
4		CMedCasual	Triple extraction	
5		CHIP-CDEE	Clinical event extraction	
6	Classification	CHIP-CTC	Criteria classification	Macro Precision,
7		KUAKE-QIC	Intent detection	Macro Recall,
8		IMCS-DAC	Intent detection	**Macro F1 scores**
9	Semantic	CHIP-STS	Disease-related questions	Micro Precision,
10	Matching	KUAKE-QTR	Query and the page title	Micro Recall,
11		KUAKE-QQR	Two medical queries	**Micro F1 Scores**
12		KUAKE-IR	Query and doc in corpus	
13		CHIP-CDN	Term Standardization	
14	Text	Med-DG	Doctor's next reply	Rouge-1, Rouge-2,
15	Generation	IMCS-MRG	Medical report generation	**Rouge-L Scores**
16	Decision Tree Generation	Text2DT	Decision tree generation	**Tree_Edit_Ratio**
17	Complex	CHIP-MDCFNPC	Extract and determine	Micro Precision,
18	Tasks	IMCS-SR	whether symptoms are negative or positive	Micro Recall, **Micro F1 Scores**

answer is limited in the given options, while for clinical trial screening criteria classification, LLMs are expected to answer "Not the above type" when the label is "others" in the original format.

Semantic Matching. For semantic matching tasks, LLMs are required to answer "similar" or "not similar", or even a more detailed degree of similarity, which is somewhat like converting the task into a binary or multi-class classification. For the term standardization task, the original requirement is given a diagnosis to find its corresponding standard diagnostic term, which is selected from more than 40,000 standard terms of ICD-10. Since it is impossible to input 40,000 words into LLM at one time, this task is transformed as: given the original diagnosis, select the matching word from several candidate ICD-10 diagnostic standard terms (many or none).

Generation. For generation tasks, text generation is a natural transformation, while the Text2DT [35] task requires LLM to extract decision trees from medical texts. The latter is challenging for LLMs due to the requirement for an in-depth understanding of medical texts and complex output forms.

Complex Tasks. The IMCS-SR and CHIP-MDCFNPC tasks are classified as complex tasks because they contain multiple sub-steps. First, medical entities need to be extracted from the text, which involves information extraction.

Then the extracted entities need to be converted to standard terms, and finally the entity attribute should be determined from multiple classes, which refers to multi-class classification.

3.3 Overall Score

The metrics of each task are also listed in Table 1, and F1 (micro/macro), Rouge-L, and decision tree edit ratio are considered as the main metrics in each task. To evaluate the performance of the LLMs on the whole benchmark, the overall score $Score_{overall}$ is used to calculate the final result, which is the average score of the main metric in each task, denoted as:

$$Score_{overall} = \frac{\sum_i^N Score_{main}^i}{N}, \tag{1}$$

where N is the number of tasks in the benchmark, and $Score_{main}^i$ is the score of main metric in task i.

4 CMed-Baichuan Model

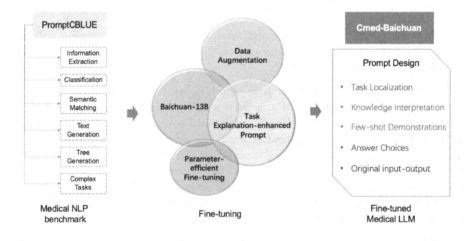

Fig. 1. The whole training process of our proposed CMed-Baichuan. The four key parts of fine-tuning are introduced from Sects. 4.1 to 4.4.

In this section, we will introduce the training process and key components of our CMed-Baichuan model, including the base model, data augmentation, efficient fine-tuning on open-source LLMs, and the details for construct prompts. Figure 1 illustrates an overview of this process.

4.1   Base Model

Baichuan LLMs [1], is a series of open source and commercially available large-scale language models with parameters ranging from 7 billion to 13 billion. It achieves promising performance among same-sized models in authoritative Chinese and English benchmarks. Here, we adopted the Baichuan-13B-chat as the base model for more accessible training.

4.2   Data Augmentation

The PromptCBLUE benchmark is obtained by transforming CBLUE tasks into prompt-based language generation tasks. However, the PromptCBLUE benchmark only occupies a portion of the original CBLUE [33] data, resulting in a reduction in the total amount of samples and dilution of few-shot samples. For medical tasks, the distribution of data itself is imbalanced, so it is more sensitive to the reduction of data volume. Therefore, we choose to use data augmentation to artificially increase training data by generating new data points from existing data. Specifically, we use direct transformation and indirect transformation to randomly sample a subset from the original CBLUE dataset for data augmentation.

Direct Transformation. Direct transformation encompasses the implementation of prompt design, as elucidated in Sect. 4.4, to randomly choose distinct sub-tasks from CBLUE and control the chosen data through prompt manipulation. This process modifies the original data to produce fresh and varied iterations.

Indirect Transformation. On the contrary, indirect transformation does not hinge on direct conversion employing CBLUE data. For example, the KUAKE-IR subtask, originally part of the CBLUE, is an information retrieval task. It involves retrieving relevant documents from a corpus of over 1 million documents based on a search query, which has a high computational complexity and large data volume, making it difficult to complete without using external vector databases or models. To address this challenge, the PromptCBLUE benchmark simplified the task by converting it into a binary classification problem. Pairs of queries and documents were randomly sampled to create individual samples, and the relevance between the query and the document was determined. This transformation represents an instance of indirect transformation.

Due to the uneven distribution of data samples across sub-tasks in the original CBLUE dataset, the application of data augmentation results in a varying distribution of PromptCBLUE data across different sub-tasks. This disparity in distribution implies that tasks with smaller datasets have a lower probability of being effectively trained and learned by the model, thus compromising their accuracy as well as the accuracy of other sub-tasks. Subsequent chapters will focus on investigating the consequences of this observation through upsampling experiments.

4.3 Parameter-Efficient Fine-Tuning

Due to the substantial parameter size and high training costs associated with large language models (LLMs), initiating the training of such models from scratch demands a considerable amount of time and financial investment, resulting in significantly low cost-effectiveness. Consequently, fine-tuning stands as an exceedingly efficient approach to enhancing the capabilities of large language models within specific domains. In terms of parameter scale, fine-tuning for large language models primarily follows two technical paths: one entails comprehensive training of all parameters, known as Full Fine Tuning (FFT), while the other selectively trains only certain parameters, referred to as Parameter-Efficient Fine Tuning (PEFT). From the perspective of training data sources and methodologies, the fine-tuning paths for large models are categorized into Supervised Fine Tuning (SFT), Reinforcement Learning with Human Feedback (RLHF), and Reinforcement Learning with AI Feedback (RLAIF). Regardless of classification, the ultimate aim of fine-tuning is to enhance the abilities of large models in specific domains while maintaining manageable costs.

Considering cost and effectiveness, PEFT represents the currently favored fine-tuning approach. This includes methodologies such as Prompt Tuning, Prefix Tuning, Low Rank Adapters (LoRA), and notably, QLoRA. Particularly, QLoRA serves as an effective fine-tuning method that significantly reduces training costs while preserving model efficacy. It is capable of fine-tuning a 65B parameter model on a single 48 GB GPU by utilizing a frozen 4-bit quantized pre-trained language model to backpropagate gradients to LoRA [5].

Thus, in this paper, we employ the QLoRA method to fine-tune the Baichuan-13B-Chat model. The additional parameter volume in parameter-efficient fine-tuning modules does not exceed 1% of the primary parameter volume of the large model's backbone.

4.4 Task Explanation-Enhanced Prompt

Prompt engineering holds a pivotal position in the realm of the Large Language Model, similar to the significance of feature engineering in the domain of machine learning. Prompt engineering, similar to feature engineering, involves the manual manipulation of input data at the model's input layer, with the objective of enhancing the model's ability to extract informative and effective information from the input data. They all serve as direct and efficient means to enhance the performance of the network model.

In the context of GPT-NER [25], the prompt is designed in three parts: Task Description, Few-shot Demonstration, and Input Sentence. The Task Description provides an overview of the input assignment, which involves informing the model of the required role, describing the task in detail, and identifying the categories of entities to be extracted from each input sentence. The Few-shot Demonstration presents the task through exemplary representations, text alignment using unique symbols, and describing the input-output format. The last section of the prompt focuses on the input of specific training instances.

However, the prompt in GPT-NER is tailored towards specific named entity recognition tasks, whereas promptCBLUE encompasses multi-task data across 18 categories. The prompt in GPT-NER necessitates the development of expansions and refinements to address specific multi-tasking challenges.

The original PromptCBLUE comprises 18 sub-tasks, with each sub-task featuring a distinct prompt aimed at enhancing the model's resilience and providing improved responses to diverse inputs. A total of 450 unique prompt templates were designed for these 18 sub-tasks, enabling a more effective activation of the model's knowledge gained from the training data. In tasks such as classification, named entity recognition (NER), and information extraction (IE), prompt templates typically consist of commands, input text, and answer choices. Among these components, answer choices serve as a constraint on the output results. For instance, in the NER subtask, the output is restricted to a specific answer choice from a pre-defined set. In the creation of sub-tasks, the structure of prompts also includes explanations for the input and introductions to medical knowledge. For instance, in the Text2DT sub-task, the prompt encompasses clarifications regarding the condition nodes and decision nodes of a binary decision tree, along with formatting instructions for the binary decision tree.

The original prompt is already endowed with the essential abilities to be fine-tuned by large language models and activate downstream tasks. Furthermore, after fine-tuning, no hallucination phenomenon occurred in the model, and it has already exhibited a certain level of robustness. Initially, In the design of multi-task prompts, it is not feasible to visually discern the variations between sub-tasks, nor can one precisely ascertain the corresponding sub-task through the prompt. Thus, prompts lack task-localization information. Additionally, the original prompt lacks a comprehensive description of the model's role, including specific terminologies, scenarios, and modes of expression. Afterward, some medical terms are difficult to comprehend at face value, including the term "chief complaint," which denotes the patient's primary and most distressing symptoms and serves as the main reason for seeking medical attention. The original prompt lacked an expository explanation of these technical terminologies, potentially contributing to the model's inadequate performance during fine-tuning due to its failure to comprehend the input terminologies. Finally, The original prompt lacks representative examples of specific samples for each sub-task.

As shown in Fig. 2, we structured the prompt design into five parts: Task Localization, Knowledge Interpretation, Few-shot Demonstrations, Answer Choices, and Original input-output.

Task Localization. The first part of the prompt is Task Localization. The prompt begins with Task Localization, whose primary objective is to precisely guide the input to a designated sub-task within the multi-task paradigm through a meticulously crafted prompt. This not only enables the model to expeditiously zero in on the designated sub-task for training and inference but also minimizes cross-talk and interference with other concurrent sub-tasks. Task Localization can be further segregated into two components:

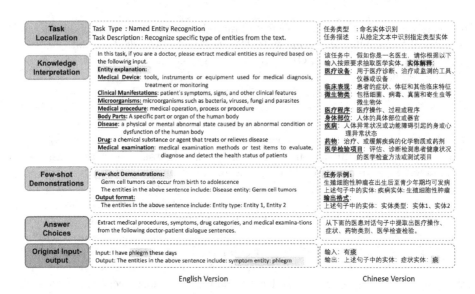

Task Localization	Task Type : Named Entity Recognition Task Description : Recognize specific type of entities from the text.	任务类型 ：命名实体识别 任务描述 ：从给定文本中识别指定类型实体
Knowledge Interpretation	In this task, if you are a doctor, please extract medical entities as required based on the following input. **Entity explanation:** **Medical Device:** tools, instruments or equipment used for medical diagnosis, treatment or monitoring **Clinical Manifestations:** patient's symptoms, signs, and other clinical features **Microorganisms:** microorganisms such as bacteria, viruses, fungi and parasites **Medical procedure:** medical operation, process or procedure **Body Parts:** A specific part or organ of the human body **Disease:** a physical or mental abnormal state caused by an abnormal condition or dysfunction of the human body **Drug:** a chemical substance or agent that treats or relieves disease **Medical examination:** medical examination methods or test items to evaluate, diagnose and detect the health status of patients	该任务中，假如你是一名医生，请你根据以下输入按照要求抽取医学实体。**实体解释：** **医疗设备：** 用于医疗诊断、治疗或监测的工具、仪器或设备 **临床表现：** 患者的症状、体征和其他临床特征 **微生物类：** 包括细菌、病毒、真菌和寄生虫等微生物体 **医疗程序：** 医疗操作、过程或程序 **身体部位：** 人体的具体部位或器官 **疾病：** 人体异常状况或功能障碍引起的身或心理异常状态 **药物：** 治疗、或缓解疾病的化学物质或药剂 **医学检验项目：** 评估、诊断检测患者健康状况的医学检查方法或测试项目
Few-shot Demonstrations	**Few-shot Demonstrations:** Germ cell tumors can occur from birth to adolescence The entities in the above sentence include: Disease entity: Germ cell tumors **Output format:** The entities in the above sentence include: Entity type: Entity 1, Entity 2	**任务示例：** 生殖细胞性肿瘤在出生至青少年期均可发病 上述句子中的实体：疾病实体：生殖细胞性肿瘤 **输出格式：** 上述句子中的实体：实体类型：实体1、实体2
Answer Choices	Extract medical procedures, symptoms, drug categories, and medical examina-tions from the following doctor-patient dialogue sentences.	从下面的医患对话句子中提取出医疗操作、症状、药物类别、医学检查检验。
Original Input-output	Input: I have phlegm these days Output: The entities in the above sentence include: symptom entity: phlegm	输入：有痰 输出：上述句子中的实体：症状实体：痰

English Version   Chinese Version

Fig. 2. Prompt Design. The details for the five parts are listed in both the English version and the Chinese version.

(1) Task Type

The Task Type specifies the type of task the sample data is associated with, such as classification, named entity recognition, information extraction, or generation tasks. Identifying a clear task type can aid the model in developing a distinct understanding and processing of the subsequent data.

(2) Task Description

The Task Description offers detailed accounts of the specifics of the task, the approaches, and the objectives related to the sample data.

Knowledge Interpretation. While general large language models lack the injection of domain-specific medical knowledge and the activation of domain-specific abilities, directly using medical domain-specific data for fine-tuning may not guarantee that the model fully understands medical terms. Therefore, adding detailed explanations of medical-specific terms can further activate the model's emergent abilities in the medical domain. An example of a specific explanation is the "Clinical manifestations: symptoms, signs, and other clinical characteristics of patients". A further aspect of Knowledge Interpretation is the suggestion of a role for the model to play, which can restrict the model's knowledge base and establish the style of its answer, thus increasing its understanding of the prompt.

Few-Shot Demonstrations. Apart from enabling the model to acquire in-depth knowledge about specific subtasks, providing concrete few-shot examples also governs the model's actual output. In the CHIP-PromptCBLUE task, with the exception of three generation tasks including MedDG, IMCS-V2-MRG, and Text2DT, the evaluation of the remaining subtasks strictly adheres to precision, recall, and F1 metrics. Only precise reasoning can be considered as accurate results. Large language models often yield unstable inference outcomes that require post-processing scripts to convert their output into accurate results. The official evaluation script converts outcomes based on a fixed template that includes pre-defined text and punctuation marks. Therefore, prompts must exercise strict control over formatting. Besides providing few-shot examples, we have also abstracted formatting requirements for different subtasks' inference results. For instance, "Output format: The entities stated in the above sentence comprise: Entity type: Entity 1, Entity 2." Furthermore, punctuation marks in both Chinese and English versions must be used with precision.

Answer Choices. Answer choices denote the entities and classification options of the reasoning outcomes in classification, named entity recognition, and information extraction tasks, constraining the model to select from the correct results. For instance, "Extract medical procedures, symptoms, drug identification, and medical tests and inspections from the following doctor-patient conversation sentence".

5 Experiment

5.1 Baselines

To have a better comparison, we choose three open-source LLMs as baselines.

ChatGLM2-6B. ChatGLM2-6B, the second-generation version of the ChatGLM-6B conversational AI developed by the Knowledge Engineering Group (KEG) & Data Mining at Tsinghua University, inherits the smooth dialogue and ease of deployment from its predecessor. It introduces enhancements such as improved performance, longer context understanding, more efficient inference, and a more open protocol. These improvements significantly enhance its capabilities in performance, context length, inference speed, and weight utilization, granting it strong competitiveness and extensive potential applications in handling conversations and processing extremely long contexts. The model version utilized in our experiments is "ChatGLM2-6B."

Llama2-Chinese-13B-Chat. Llama 2 is Meta's first open-source commercially available large language model, pre-trained on 20 trillion tokens and fine-tuned on 1 million human-labeled data to create a conversational model. It significantly outperforms open-source large language models such as MPT, Falcon, and the first-generation LLaMA in many benchmarks, including inference, programming, conversation, and knowledge testing. Llama2-Chinese-13B is the Chinese version of the 13B Llama2 model, significantly enhancing and optimizing Llama2's Chinese capabilities at the model's core. The model version utilized in our experiments is "Llama2-Chinese-13B."

Baichuan-13B-Chat. Baichuan-13B [1], an open-source commercially available large-scale language model developed by Baichuan Intelligence, contains 13 billion parameters. It achieves promising performance among same-sized models in authoritative Chinese and English benchmarks. This release includes two versions: pre-trained (Baichuan-13B-Base), which lacks alignment with human preferences and cannot engage in direct conversation, and aligned (Baichuan-13B-Chat), which aligns with human preferences, enabling direct conversation. The model version utilized in our experiments is "Baichuan-13B-Chat."

5.2   Hyper-Parameters and Environment

We fine-tuned CMed-Baichuan 4 epochs on PromptCBLUE with per device batch size 4, gradient accumulation 4, and learning rate 2e−4. All experiments were done on a single NVIDIA 4090 GPU (24 GB).

5.3   Results

We evaluate CMed-Baichuan on the PromptCBLUE benchmark. The results are reported in Table 2. Our fine-tuned LLM achieves state-of-art performance on the average score on 18 tasks, where achieves the best performance in 13 tasks, and competitive performance on the rest 5 tasks.

Table 2. The results of CMed-Baichuan on 18 medical benchmarks. (**Bold**: the best; <u>Underline</u>: the second best)

Benchmark	Metrics	Chatglm2-6B	Llama-13B	Baichuan-13B	CMed-Baichuan
CMeEE	Micro-F1	65.4989	65.9596	67.1391	**67.5676**
CMeIE	Micro-F1	35.3116	**41.2553**	37.5967	40.6020
CHIP-CDN	Micro-F1	74.4917	76.9103	79.8182	**86.2229**
CHIP-CDEE	Micro-F1	57.8947	**61.7949**	61.7857	**61.7450**
IMCS-NER	Micro-F1	82.9224	85.3492	85.4299	**86.9863**
CHIP-MDCFNPC	Micro-F1	61.8174	73.4459	65.3775	**76.1847**
IMCS-SR	Micro-F1	70.3767	73.4443	72.6496	**73.8786**
IMCS-DAC	Macro-F1	69.5923	69.7844	**78.8152**	78.7728
CHIP-CTC	Macro-F1	63.0877	**72.7356**	71.2843	69.3533
CHIP-STS	Micro-F1	81.4819	75.9342	82.4829	**82.5092**
KUAKE-IR	Micro-F1	84.3079	85.3360	86.7181	**87.8221**
KUAKE-QIC	Macro-F1	91.2786	90.0445	92.1512	**92.6134**
KUAKE-QQR	Micro-F1	74.6385	74.2286	**78.0232**	77.0817
KUAKE-QTR	Micro-F1	61.8431	60.2588	62.8472	**66.4198**
MedDG	RougeL	9.1517	8.5922	**9.6526**	8.5267
Text2DT	TreeLenvRatio	80.5399	77.4051	79.5623	**82.4020**
CMedCausal	Micro-F1	31.2683	36.6323	**38.8171**	37.7818
IMCS-MRG	RougeL	45.4901	47.3447	48.1425	**49.1475**
Score		63.3885	65.3587	66.5718	**68.0899**

5.4   Parameter Optimization

In parameter optimization, the initial parameters that should be adjusted are the learning rate and step. A low learning rate may result in underfitting of the model, while a high learning rate may lead to overfitting. Additionally, different learning rates correspond to different step sizes for achieving optimal model performance. For example, a lower learning rate corresponds to a longer step size for achieving good model performance, but a step size that is too long may increase the training time cost and make it difficult to train a satisfactory model within a limited time frame. Therefore, we begin with the default learning rate of 5e−5 and use a maximum training step size of 61000 to determine the optimal learning rate and corresponding step for different models.

Table 3. Performance of the best score and corresponding step under different learning rates and a maximum step of 61,000.

Learning rate	Best score	Steps
5e−5	59.15	61000
1e−4	62.25	61000
2e−4	64.95	20000

Table 3 demonstrates that when the learning rates are 5e−5 and 1e−4, the model achieves its best performance on the validation set at the maximum training step. However, the excessive training time required for reaching the maximum step of 61000 makes it challenging to iterate toward an even better performance within a limited time using these learning rates as the baseline. Although there might be a slight possibility of attaining an even better score after the maximum training step for learning rates of 5e−5 and 1e−4, considering the excessive training costs, we decided to continue increasing the learning rate instead. Consequently, we tested a larger learning rate of 2e−4 and observed the optimal score at approximately step 20000.

As reported in Fig. 3, for a learning rate of 2e−4, the score reached its peak at step 20000 and then gradually declined, indicating an overfitting state. This step roughly corresponds to epoch 4, which represents a balance point between the learning rate and training time that we identified. An overly large learning rate might lead to oscillations during the optimization process and prevent the model from converging to a stable solution. Therefore, we ultimately selected a learning rate of 2e−4 and determined the optimal step based on specific data and prompt experiments at around 20000 steps.

5.5   Analysis on Data Augmentation

As shown in Table 4, "original" refers to the prediction results of the baichuan model on various benchmarks at epoch 1, whereas "augmentation" signifies the

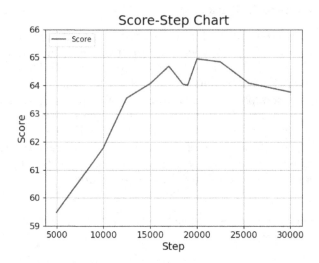

Fig. 3. The overall score with the learning rate at 2e−4 in the training process. The x-axis is the training step.

Table 4. The results of augmentation without upsampling on 18 medical benchmarks.

Benchmark	Metrics	original	augmentation	delta
CMeEE	Micro-F1	64.4786	65.4314	+0.9528
CMeIE	Micro-F1	38.1797	38.3749	+0.1952
CHIP-CDN	Micro-F1	77.6860	78.0988	+0.4128
CHIP-CDEE	Micro-F1	61.9990	62.3244	+0.3254
IMCS-NER	Micro-F1	82.5112	83.6036	+1.0924
CHIP-MDCFNPC	Micro-F1	65.9504	66.2263	+0.2759
IMCS-SR	Micro-F1	70.3959	71.9178	+1.5219
IMCS-DAC	Macro-F1	76.7846	77.4008	+0.6162
CHIP-CTC	Macro-F1	71.5548	73.9559	+2.4010
CHIP-STS	Micro-F1	82.2119	83.2369	+1.0250
KUAKE-IR	Micro-F1	84.0750	82.7085	−1.3665
KUAKE-QIC	Macro-F1	91.7995	92.1513	+0.3518
KUAKE-QQR	Micro-F1	78.3942	77.1468	−1.2473
KUAKE-QTR	Micro-F1	60.9784	59.6433	−1.3351
MedDG	RougeL	9.2863	8.7352	−0.5511
Text2DT	TreeLenvRatio	80.5370	79.3090	−1.2280
CMedCausal	Micro-F1	38.9205	38.0144	−0.9061
IMCS-MRG	RougeL	49.3309	47.6872	−1.6437
Score		65.8374	65.8870	+0.0495

results of implementing an extra 20% data augmentation on the CMeEE and CHIP-STS subtasks within the training data without upsampling, followed by predictions again at epoch 1 of the baichuan model. "delta" represents the difference in metric values between "augmentation" and "original". The two subtasks that undergo data augmentation experience a metric increase of approximately 1%, affirming the efficacy of data augmentation. However, among the remaining subtasks, the metrics of 9 subtasks improve, while the metrics of 7 subtasks decline. Overall, the metric only improves by 0.01%, which can be considered minimal. While enhancing the performance of some tasks may result in an increase in the metrics of other tasks, enhancing the data volume of some subtasks by 20% may lead to a decrease in the proportion of other subtasks, particularly non-homologous subtasks. This decrease may contribute to a reduction in the model's training samples for these subtasks. Therefore, it emphasizes the importance of upsampling.

6   Case Study

Figure 4 illustrates the case performances of various models across the CMeEE, CHIP-MDCFNPC, and CHIP-CDN tasks. These examples contribute to a more intuitive understanding of how different models handle tasks and aid in evaluating their capabilities.

6.1   CMeEE

As shown in Fig. 4(a), within the CMeEE task, the CMED model exhibited flawless entity recognition abilities in the provided examples. Compared to Baichuan and LLaMA, CMED accurately identified medical procedure entities like "staining" and microbial entities like "bacteria," ensuring precise annotations of entity boundaries and types. This highlights CMED's exceptional capacity in comprehending text contexts and accurately identifying entities and their categories.

6.2   CHIP-MDCFNPC

As depicted in Fig. 4(b), in this task, although CMED had one annotation error (labeling the "hepatic function abnormality" entity, categorized as "positive," as "unlabeled"), its overall performance remained more accurate compared to other models. With lower error rates than Baichuan and LLaMA, CMED demonstrated a better understanding and classification capability regarding clinical entity positive/negative labels.

6.3   CHIP-CDN

As illustrated in Fig. 4(c), in the CHIP-CDN task, models are required to convert original diagnostic descriptions into matching standard terms, ensuring correct

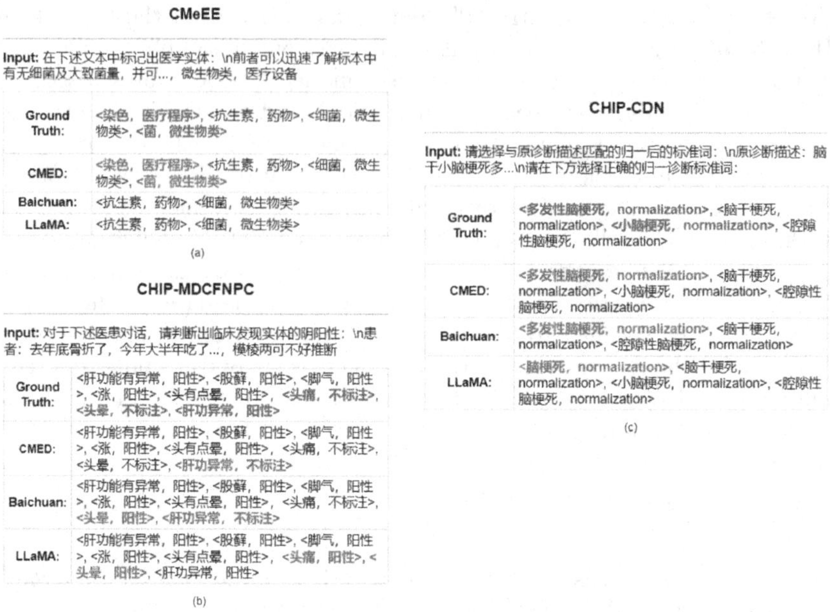

CMeEE

Input: 在下述文本中标记出医学实体: \n前者可以迅速了解标本中有无细菌及大致菌量, 并可..., 微生物类, 医疗设备

Ground Truth:	<染色, 医疗程序>, <抗生素, 药物>, <细菌, 微生物类>, <菌, 微生物类>
CMED:	<染色, 医疗程序>, <抗生素, 药物>, <细菌, 微生物类>, <菌, 微生物类>
Baichuan:	<抗生素, 药物>, <细菌, 微生物类>
LLaMA:	<抗生素, 药物>, <细菌, 微生物类>

(a)

CHIP-MDCFNPC

Input: 对于下述医患对话, 请判断出临床发现实体的阴阳性: \n患者: 去年底骨折了, 今年大半年吃了..., 模棱两可不好推断

Ground Truth:	<肝功能有异常, 阳性>, <股藓, 阳性>, <脚气, 阳性>, <涨, 阳性>, <头有点晕, 阳性>, <头痛, 不标注>, <头晕, 不标注>, <肝功异常, 阳性>
CMED:	<肝功能有异常, 阳性>, <股藓, 阳性>, <脚气, 阳性>, <涨, 阳性>, <头有点晕, 阳性>, <头痛, 不标注>, <头晕, 不标注>, <肝功异常, 不标注>
Baichuan:	<肝功能有异常, 阳性>, <股藓, 阳性>, <脚气, 阳性>, <涨, 阳性>, <头有点晕, 阳性>, <头痛, 不标注>, <头晕, 阳性>, <肝功异常, 不标注>
LLaMA:	<肝功能有异常, 阳性>, <股藓, 阳性>, <脚气, 阳性>, <涨, 阳性>, <头有点晕, 阳性>, <头痛, 阳性>, <头晕, 阳性>, <肝功异常, 阳性>

(b)

CHIP-CDN

Input: 请选择与原诊断描述匹配的归一后的标准词: \n原诊断描述: 脑干小脑梗死多...\n请在下方选择正确的归一诊断标准词:

Ground Truth:	<多发性脑梗死, normalization>, <脑干梗死, normalization>, <小脑梗死, normalization>, <腔隙性脑梗死, normalization>
CMED:	<多发性脑梗死, normalization>, <脑干梗死, normalization>, <小脑梗死, normalization>, <腔隙性脑梗死, normalization>
Baichuan:	<多发性脑梗死, normalization>, <脑干梗死, normalization>, <腔隙性脑梗死, normalization>
LLaMA:	<脑梗死, normalization>, <脑干梗死, normalization>, <小脑梗死, normalization>, <腔隙性脑梗死, normalization>

(c)

Fig. 4. Cases of on the CMeEE, CHIP-CDN and CHIP-MDCFNPC tasks.

and complete term matches. The CMED model displayed entirely accurate annotations, whereas the Baichuan model omitted the term "cerebellar infarction," and the LLaMA model omitted the label "multiple cerebral infarctions" and incorrectly labeled it as "cerebral infarction."

Overall, across these three tasks, the CMED model showcased outstanding performance in entity recognition, classification, and standard term matching. Though not flawless, relative to other comparative models, CMED exhibited higher accuracy and stability in these tasks, demonstrating superior overall performance.

7   Conclusion

In this paper, we studied the evaluation of large language models in the PromptCBLUE benchmark and proposed a task explanation-enhanced medical LLM (CMed-Baichuan). Specifically, we first applied data augmentation on each task dataset. Next, we proposed the task-based prompting method to improve the LLM's understanding of the requirements of task and instruction. Furthermore, we demonstrated the effectiveness of task explanation and evaluated the performance of three public LLMs and our fine-tuned CMed-Baichuan through extensive experiments on 18 medical tasks. The results showed that our model achieves state-of-the-art overall performance, where achieves best performance in 13 tasks, and competitive performance on the rest 5 tasks.

In the future, we hope to further explore the interpretability of the medical LLMs, which is vital to the medical domain. The current challenge lies in the inherent lack of transparency and interpretability, hindering the seamless integration of LLMs into medical tasks. Addressing this challenge is imperative to unlock the full potential of large models in assisting healthcare professionals and patients in practical scenarios.

References

1. Baichuan: Baichuan 2: Open large-scale language models. arXiv preprint arXiv:2309.10305 (2023)
2. Brown, T.B., et al.: Language models are few-shot learners (2020)
3. Chang, Y., et al.: A survey on evaluation of large language models. arXiv (2023). https://doi.org/10.48550/arxiv.2307.03109
4. Chowdhery, A., et al.: PaLM: scaling language modeling with pathways. arXiv (2022). https://doi.org/10.48550/arxiv.2204.02311
5. Dettmers, T., Pagnoni, A., Holtzman, A., Zettlemoyer, L.: QLoRA: efficient fine-tuning of quantized LLMs. arXiv (2023)
6. Du, Z., et al.: GLM: general language model pretraining with autoregressive blank infilling. In: Proceedings of the 60th Annual Meeting of the Association for Computational Linguistics (Volume 1: Long Papers), pp. 320–335 (2022)
7. Floridi, L., Chiriatti, M.: GPT-3: its nature, scope, limits, and consequences. Mind. Mach. **30**(4), 681–694 (2020). https://doi.org/10.1007/s11023-020-09548-1
8. Gekhman, Z., Herzig, J., Aharoni, R., Elkind, C., Szpektor, I.: TrueTeacher: learning factual consistency evaluation with large language models. arXiv (2023). https://doi.org/10.48550/arxiv.2305.11171
9. Hu, E.J., et al.: LoRA: low-rank adaptation of large language models. In: International Conference on Learning Representations (2022). https://openreview.net/forum?id=nZeVKeeFYf9
10. Kamalloo, E., Dziri, N., Clarke, C.L.A., Rafiei, D.: Evaluating open-domain question answering in the era of large language models (2023)
11. Lester, B., Al-Rfou, R., Constant, N.: The power of scale for parameter-efficient prompt tuning (2021)
12. Li, J., Li, R., Liu, Q.: Beyond static datasets: a deep interaction approach to LLM evaluation. arXiv (2023). https://doi.org/10.48550/arxiv.2309.04369
13. Li, X.L., Liang, P.: Prefix-tuning: optimizing continuous prompts for generation (2021)
14. Li, X., et al.: Unified demonstration retriever for in-context learning (2023)
15. Liu, X., et al.: P-tuning v2: prompt tuning can be comparable to fine-tuning universally across scales and tasks (2022)
16. OpenAI: GPT-4 technical report (2023)
17. Ouyang, L., et al.: Training language models to follow instructions with human feedback (2022)
18. Power, A., Burda, Y., Edwards, H., Babuschkin, I., Misra, V.: Grokking: generalization beyond overfitting on small algorithmic datasets. arXiv (2022). https://doi.org/10.48550/arxiv.2201.02177
19. Qin, G., Eisner, J.: Learning how to ask: querying LMs with mixtures of soft prompts. In: Toutanova, K., et al. (eds.) Proceedings of the 2021 Conference

of the North American Chapter of the Association for Computational Linguistics: Human Language Technologies, pp. 5203–5212. Association for Computational Linguistics, Online (2021). https://doi.org/10.18653/v1/2021.naacl-main.410. https://aclanthology.org/2021.naacl-main.410

20. Shin, T., Razeghi, Y., Logan, R.L., IV., Wallace, E., Singh, S.: Autoprompt: eliciting knowledge from language models with automatically generated prompts (2020)
21. Singhal, K., et al.: Large language models encode clinical knowledge. Nature **620**(7972), 172–180 (2023). https://doi.org/10.1038/s41586-023-06291-2
22. Sun, F.K., Lai, C.I.: Conditioned natural language generation using only unconditioned language model: an exploration (2020)
23. Touvron, H., et al.: LLaMA: open and efficient foundation language models (2023)
24. Touvron, H., et al.: LLaMA 2: open foundation and fine-tuned chat models (2023)
25. Wang, S., et al.: GPT-NER: named entity recognition via large language models (2023)
26. Wang, Y., et al.: PandaLM: an automatic evaluation benchmark for LLM instruction tuning optimization. arXiv (2023). https://doi.org/10.48550/arxiv.2306.05087
27. Wei, J., et al.: Finetuned language models are zero-shot learners (2022)
28. Wei, J., et al.: Emergent abilities of large language models. arXiv (2022). https://doi.org/10.48550/arxiv.2206.07682
29. Wen, Y., Jain, N., Kirchenbauer, J., Goldblum, M., Geiping, J., Goldstein, T.: Hard prompts made easy: gradient-based discrete optimization for prompt tuning and discovery (2023)
30. Yang, J., et al.: Harnessing the power of LLMs in practice: a survey on ChatGPT and beyond (2023)
31. Zeng, A., et al.: GLM-130B: an open bilingual pre-trained model. arXiv preprint arXiv:2210.02414 (2022)
32. Zhang, H., et al.: HuatuoGPT, towards taming language model to be a doctor. arXiv (2023). https://doi.org/10.48550/arxiv.2305.15075
33. Zhang, N., et al.: CBLUE: a Chinese biomedical language understanding evaluation benchmark. In: Muresan, S., Nakov, P., Villavicencio, A. (eds.) Proceedings of the 60th Annual Meeting of the Association for Computational Linguistics, Dublin, Ireland (Volume 1: Long Papers), pp. 7888–7915. Association for Computational Linguistics (2022). https://doi.org/10.18653/v1/2022.acl-long.544. https://aclanthology.org/2022.acl-long.544
34. Zhang, S., et al.: OPT: open pre-trained transformer language models. arXiv (2022). https://doi.org/10.48550/arxiv.2205.01068
35. Zhu, W., et al.: Extracting decision trees from medical texts: an overview of the Text2DT track in CHIP2022. In: Tang, B., et al. (eds.) Health Information Processing. Evaluation Track Papers, vol. 1773, pp. 89–102. Springer, Singapore (2023). https://doi.org/10.1007/978-981-99-4826-0_9
36. Zhu, W., Wang, X., Chen, M., Tang, B.: Overview of the PromptCBLUE shared task in CHIP2023 (2023)
37. Zhu, W., Wang, X., Zheng, H., Chen, M., Tang, B.: PromptCBLUE: a Chinese prompt tuning benchmark for the medical domain (2023)
38. Zhu, W., et al.: Multilingual machine translation with large language models: empirical results and analysis. arXiv (2023). https://doi.org/10.48550/arxiv.2304.04675

Improving LLM-Based Health Information Extraction with In-Context Learning

Junkai Liu, Jiayi Wang, Hui Huang, Rui Zhang, Muyun Yang$^{(\boxtimes)}$, and Tiejun Zhao

Research Center on Language Technology, School of Computer Science and Engineering, Harbin Institute of Technology, Harbin, China
{7203610511,2021111542,huanghui,23S003048}@stu.hit.edu.cn,
{yangmuyun,tjzhao}@hit.edu.cn

Abstract. The Large Language Model (LLM) has received widespread attention in the industry. In the context of the popularity of LLM, almost all NLP tasks are transformed into prompt based language generation tasks. On the other hand, LLM can also achieve superior results on brand new tasks without fine-tuning, solely with a few in-context examples. This paper describes our participation in the China Health Information Processing Conference (CHIP 2023). We focused on in-context learning (ICL) and experimented with different combinations of demonstration retrieval strategies on the given task and tested the optimal strategy combination proposed by us. The experimental results show that our retrieval strategies based on Chinese-LlaMA2-13B-chat achieved a average score of 40.27, ranked the first place among five teams, confirmed the effectiveness of our method.

Keywords: Large Language Model · Health Information Extraction · In-context Learning

1 Introduction

In the past, NLP engineers were accustomed to finetuning a pretrained model on a task-specific in a fully-supervised manner. Both the collection of datasets and the finetuning of pretrained models are quite resource intensive, sometimes hard to implement [1]. Until recently, large language models (LLMs), with powerful generation capabilities, could be applied in any existing task or a brand new one by transform it into a prompt based language generation task.

Chinese Biomedical Language Understanding Evaluation (CBLUE) benchmark is a collection of natural language understanding tasks including named entity recognition, information extraction, clinical diagnosis normalization, and an associated online platform for model evaluation, comparison, and analysis [2]. The non fine-tuning track we participate in requires that the parameters of the LLM cannot be modified. Integrate with multi-LLMs or extract information based on multi-round interaction is also not allowed. Therefore, the main source of performance improvement in the evaluation will be the improvement of demonstration retrieval.

This paper put forward a set of methods for better demonstration retrieval. Our methodology divides the retrieval pipeline into three stages: scoring (grade every candidate demonstration), combining (select demonstrations from candidate set to build prompt) and ranking (rank selected demonstrations with certain order). This pipeline would build a high-quality prompt, enabling the LLM functions to be a better information extractor. We experimented different LLMs and retrieval strategy combinations of the three stages on the evaluation benchmark and determined an optimal combination using Chinese-LlaMA2-13B-chat, which achieved an average score of 40.27 in final test dataset, near the score 42.03 got by ChatGPT using baseline ICL method [2]. Additionally, we also experimented with probability calibration that were not integrated into the final result due to competition rules.

2   Related Work

2.1   Large Language Model and In-Context Learning

LLM refers to language models based on transformer architecture containing hundreds of billions (or more) of parameters, which are trained on large-scale textual data, such as GPT-3 [3], PaLM [4], Galactica [5], and LLaMA [6]. LLMs have demonstrated the powerful ability to understand natural language and solve complex tasks through text generation. As they are pre-trained on a mixture of source corpora, they can capture rich knowledge from large-scale pre-training data, thus having the potential to serve as domain experts or specialists for specific areas. Meanwhile, they could also be conveniently adapted for the domains where they could not perform well by instruction tuning [7] and alignment tuning [8]. It has been shown that LLMs are capable of facilitating a variety of healthcare, education, finance and scientific research [9].

Despite the excellent performance it has achieved, LLMs can be further improved with a simple strategy called In-context Learning [3]. In-context learning is intended to improve model performance solely by editing prompt. It uses a formatted natural language prompt, consisting of the task description and/or a few task examples as demonstrations. The reason why ICL could work is because LLMs possess the ability of few-shot, which means they could get a fine result in a brand-new task provided with several demonstration, without the need for additional training or gradient updates [3].

Regarding the underlying mechanism of ICL, LLMs generate meta gradients with respect to demonstrations and implicitly perform gradient descent via the attention mechanism by means of forward computation [10]. Previous studies have shown that only models with a certain scale of parameters have the ability of learning from demonstrations. For example, in the GPT series of language model, GPT-3 with 175B parameters has been proven to exhibit strong ICL capabilities in general situations while GPT-1 and GPT-2 not [9].

2.2   Information Extraction Based on LLM

Information Extraction (IE) aims to extract structured information from unstructured texts. It is a complex task comprised of a wide range of sub-tasks, such as named, nominal, and pronominal mention extraction, entity linking, entity coreference resolution, relation extraction, event extraction, and event coreference resolution [11]. Many studies have applied LLM to information extraction tasks and achieved superior performance: Wei et al. [12] transformed the zero-shot IE task into a multi-turn question-answering problem with a two-stage framework (ChatIE); Li et al. [13] assessed the overall ability of ChatGPT using 7 fine-grained information extraction tasks; Ji [14] proposed VicunaNER, a zero/few-shot NER framework based on the newly released open-source LLM - Vicuna; Wadhwa et al. [15] used larger language models (GPT-3 and Flan-T5 large) than considered in prior work and evaluated their performance on standard relation extraction tasks under varying levels of supervision.

3   Our Methods

3.1   Basic LLM

Four LLMs are offered for participants, and considering the significant differences in parameter quantities among these models, we take Baichuan-13B-Chat and Chinese-LlaMA2-13B-chat [6] into account.

Both models are based on LLaMA architecture, which is based on the Transformer architecture and leverages various improvements that were subsequently proposed. The original architecture is a Transformer decoder, which consists of multiple layers, each containing self-attention mechanisms and feedforward neural networks. It takes encoded input information and generates an output sequence step by step. LLaMA added an additional layer normalization after the final self-attention block. Finally, a modified initialization which accounts for the accumulation on the residual path with model depth is used [16].

The main difference between LLaMA and the original Transformer decoder lies in three folds.First, to improve the training stability, instead of normalizing the output LLaMA normalize the input of each transformer sub-layer with the RMSNorm normalizing function [17]. Second, LLaMA replace the ReLU non-linearity by the SwiGLU activation function [18] to improve the performance. Third, LLaMA remove the absolute positional embeddings, and instead, add rotary positional embeddings (RoPE) [19] at each layer of the network.

The primary architectural differences between LLaMA1 and LLaMA2 include that LLaMA2 increased context length and grouped-query attention (GQA) [6].

3.2   Prompt Format

Prompt is a natural language sequence used to instruct LLM to generate responses. The construction of prompt has a significant impact on LLM performance. Moreover, the introduction of ICL also requires a formatted natural language prompt, consisting of the task description combined with a few task examples as demonstrations.

In practice, we format the whole prompt in the order of $(x_1^d, y_1^d, ..., x_n^d, y_n^d, I, x)$ as shown in Fig. 1 [20], where x_i^d, y_i^d, I, x are the demonstration input, demonstration output, instruction and test input respectively. This aligns with the convention of problem-solving where the task is first outlined, followed by the provision of data examples, and the test input is finally provided.

```
[demonstration list]
question:[input of demonstration #1]
answer:[output of demonstration #1]
......
question:[input of demonstration #n]
answer:[output of demonstration #n]
Please answer the following questions based on the
example above:[test input]
answer:
```

Fig. 1. Prompt format for our LLM-based information extraction.

3.3 Demonstration Retrieval Strategy

We mainly focuses on three aspects of in-context demonstrations, including the scoring, combining and ranking of demonstration examples [21]. The entire process of our proposed framework is shown in the Fig. 2.

Demonstration Scoring. An in-context example that is similar to test input could be of greater help to LLM intuitively [21]. From a mathematical perspective, we can also view that as narrowing the distribution of inputs and outputs. Therefore, we use the similarity between demonstration and test input as the score. There are two categories of similarity:

- **Co-occurrence based.** The methods based on co-occurrence all calculate similarity between two sequences from their overlapping part. In our work, we chose BM25 as a representative of this type for its reliable performance [22].
- **Distributed representation based.** Transforming a text sequence to a vector in distributed presentation space is adopted for information retrieval and extraction broadly. Vector representation enables various mathematical distances to be applied to calculate similarity, such as cosine similarity, Manhatten distance and Euclidean distance. In this work, we derive the distributed sentence representation via sentence BERT. More specifically, text2vec-base-chinese-paraphrase and text2vec-base-chinese [23], two CoSENT (Cosine Sentence) models, are adopted.

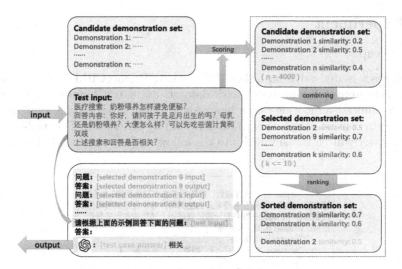

Fig. 2. An illustration of prompt construction and inference.

Demonstration Combining. Gao et al. [21] shows that there was a positive correlation between the number of demonstrations and LLM performance. Given that the LLM has a limited context window, we tried different combining methods to make the most of high-quality demonstrations within the context.

- **The greedy algorithm**. It traverse all candidate demonstrations in the order of similarity priority and append them to the prompt one by one before they exceed the context window of LLM.
- **The knapsack algorithm**. It takes the similarity of the demo as the value of the item, the length as the weight of the item, the context window size as the capacity of the knapsack, and formulate the combining process as a knapsack problem.

However, in our experiment, we found that the number of demonstration would have a negative effect to the performance when exceeding a certain level, possibly because too many demonstrations would disrupt the instruction understanding. Therefore, we set a upper-limit of 10 to the demonstration number in both combining methods.

Demonstration Ranking. The final step in building the prompt is to rank selected demonstrations in a specific order. Ranking matters whether we perform this implicit gradient descent from a higher or lower similarity. Previous work shows that arranging the demonstration examples based on their similarity to the test sample in ascending order can achieve relatively better results in most cases [21]. We take both ascending and descending order into account.

4 Experiment

4.1 Setup

The dataset is derived from CHIP 2023 task 1. PromptCBLUE, a large-scale multi-task prompt tuning benchmark dataset, evaluate Chinese LLMs' multi-task capabilities on a wide range bio-medical tasks. Over 450 instructions are provided to convert each task into the form of rely generation. The medical text NLP dataset will be transformed into the following format shown in Fig. 3.

```
{
    "input" : "医疗搜索: 奶粉喂养怎样避免便秘? \n回
答内容: 你好, 请问孩子是足月出生的吗? 母乳还是奶粉喂养?
大便怎么样? 可以先吃些茵汁黄和双歧\n上述搜索和回答是否
相关? \n选项: 相关, 不相关",
    "target" : "相关",
    "answer_choices" : [ "相关", "不相关" ],
    "task_type" : "nli",
    "task_dataset" : "KUAKE-IR",
    "sample_id" : "test-22894"
}
```

Fig. 3. A transformed example in validation set.

The tasks in PromptCBLUE [2] can be divided into the following groups:

- **Medical information extraction**, including: (a) CMeEE-V2 (medical named entity recognition), (b) CMeIE (medical triple extraction), (c) CHIP-CDEE (clinical finding event extraction), (d) CHIP-CDN, (diagnosis descriptions map), (e) IMCS-V2-NER (medical entity extraction).
- **Medical text classification**, including: (a) CHIP-CTC (Chinese eligibility criteria classification in clinical trials), (b) KUAKE-QIC (online medical queries classification), (c) IMCS-V2-DAC (medical intent classification of medical dialogues).
- **Medical natural language inference tasks**, including (a) CHIP-STS, KUAKE-QQR and KUAKE-QTR tasks (semantic relation extraction between a pair of medical queries), (b) KUAKE-IR (semantic relation extraction between a query-document pair).
- **Symptom status understanding for medical dialogues**, including IMCS-V2-SR and CHIP-MDCFNPC (clinical findings and status extraction).
- **Medical content generation**, including (a) IMCS-V2-MRG (medical dialogues summarization), (b) MedDG (generating respond to patient's queries in a dialogue).

The metrics for different tasks are shown in Table 1. It is worth mentioning that the competition does not allow modifications to instruction templates for the aim of facilitating the use of diverse templates to detect the robustness of the model.

Table 1. Evaluation metrics for different tasks

Task	Indicator
dialogue understanding	micro-F1
information extraction	micro-F1
natural language inference	micro-F1
text classification	macro-F1
content generation	ROUGE-L

4.2 Results

We experimented several combinations in dataset level. Different demonstration scoring, combining and ranking strategies, as well as different LLMs are compared. The experimental results in dataset level are shown in Table 2. Our conclusions are as follows:

Table 2. The results of different retrieval methods

LLM	Scoring	Combining	Ranking	Score
llama-13b	–	1 random	–	22.68
baichuan-13	–	1 random	–	21.11
llama-13b	BM25	greedy($= 1$)	–	26.84
llama-13b	cosine	greedy($= 1$)	–	26.59
llama-13b	BM25	greedy(≤ 5)	descending	35.05
llama-13b	BM25	greedy(≤ 12)	descending	36.20
llama-13b	cosine	greedy	descending	36.32
llama-13b	BM25	greedy	descending	36.37
llama-13b	BM25	knapsack	descending	30.61
llama-13b	Euclidean	greedy	descending	34.69
llama-13b	BM25	greedy	ascending	**36.42**
llama-13b	optimizing in task level			**40.27**
ChatGPT	ICL baseline			42.08

Table 3. The results of final submission and ChatGPT

LLM	Method	Score
llama-13b	optimizing in task level	**40.27**
ChatGPT	ICL baseline	42.08

Firstly, Llama2 performs better than baichuan by 1.5 points on the benchmark. Considering that Baichuan and Llama have similar architectures, we assume that this improvement comes from improvements such as grouped-query attention adopted by Llama 2. We also suppose that this is because more medical text is introduced in the pre-training of Llama2.

Secondly, demonstration similarity has a positive effect on in-context-learning. Comparing the result of similarity-based selection and random selection, we can see demonstrations selected by similarity has a major improvement of 4.16 points. This comes from two aspects [9]: task recognition, where similar demonstrations help LLMs recognize the task and task learning, where LLMs generate meta gradients with respect to similar demonstrations and implicitly perform gradient descent. Moreover, BM25 get the best score compared to other similarity metrics despite its simplicity. We think this is because in-context learning relies more on superficial similarity, while distributed representations such as Sentence BERT contains more semantic information. Therefore, the token co-occurence based selection functions better for in-context learning.

Moreover, The number of demonstrations would not always keep a positive correlation with performance. The score declined when increasing the upper limit from 10 to 12, demonstrating that when the number of demonstrations increased to a certain extent, the negative impact of excessively long contexts on the model outweighs the benefits from more illustration.

Last but not least, the greedy algorithm is significantly superior to knapsack algorithms in determining demonstration combination. Knapsack algorithm do not perform well and only achieved a score of 30.61, 5.76 less than greedy algorithm under the same conditions. This is because the greedy algorithm always choose the demonstrations with the highest similarity while the knapsack algorithm considers overall similarity summation. This also indicates that a small amount of high-quality demonstrations can functions better than massive low-quality demonstrations.

The above discussion are expounded in whole dataset level. But we found that the performance of different retrieval strategies varies greatly on different tasks and we managed to search for the optimal strategy combinations for different tasks. The result is shown in Table 3 and the methods for each task in our final submission are shown in Table 4.

Calibration led to significant improvements on many tasks compared to the best method. Specifically, it also achieved 4 points more than our optimal optimization on KUAKE-QTR task. The following Table 5 is the result of calibration based on BM25+greedy algorithm+descending order.

Table 4. The strategy combination for each sub-task in final submission

Task	Scoring	Combining	Ranking	Score
CMeEE-V2	BM25	greedy algorithm	descending order	35.10
CMeIE-V2	BM25	greedy algorithm	ascending order	10.09
CHIP-CDN	cos	greedy algorithm	ascending order	47.65
CHIP-CDEE	BM25	greedy algorithm	ascending order	18.33
IMCS-V2-NER	cos	greedy algorithm	descending order	61.95
CHIP-MDCFNPC	BM25	knapsack algorithm	ascending order	42.69
IMCS-V2-SR	cos	greedy algorithm	descending order	36.49
IMCS-V2-DAC	BM25	knapsack algorithm	ascending order	14.99
CHIP-CTC	cos	greedy algorithm	ascending order	62.30
CHIP-STS	cos	greedy algorithm	ascending order	73.37
KUAKE-IR	BM25	a most dissimilar demonstration	–	67.41
KUAKE-QIC	BM25	greedy algorithm	ascending order	68.03
KUAKE-QQR	cos	greedy algorithm	descending order	38.35
KUAKE-QTR	BM25	knapsack algorithm	ascending order	38.92
MedDG	BM25	greedy algorithm	descending order	13.29
TextDT	BM25	greedy algorithm	ascending order	54.41
CMedCausal	cos	greedy algorithm	descending order	6.26
IMCS-V2-MRG	BM25	knapsack algorithm	ascending order	35.14

Table 5. The result of calibration in test set

Task[a]	Non-calibration	Calibration
CHIP-CDEE	15.12	**16.21**
IMCS-V2-NER	**56.18**	54.96
CHIP-MDCFNPC	35.21	35.22
IMCS-V2-SR	30.98	**33.29**
IMCS-V2-MRG	32.29	32.29
KUAKE-IR	57.61	**68.24**
KUAKE-QQR	29.20	**42.95**
KUAKE-QTR	31.30	**33.57**

[a] All tasks were evaluated using BM25 to score, greedy algorithm to combine and ranked in descending order.

4.3 Probability Calibration

In our experiments, we also conducted calibration [24] despite prohibited by rules. Calibration aims to correct the original bias of the model. Concretely, the model's bias towards certain answers is estimated by feeding in a dummy test input that is content-free. In the absence of bias in the model, the probability of outputting each option for the null problem should be the same while LLM would be more inclined to output certain options because of bias. Therefore, we can use the difference between the model output probability and the mean to calibrate. p_b is the probability that model output a specific option with content-free input and p_o is the original probability with test input, the calibrated probability is calculated as $p_c = p_o/p_b$. The format of content-free input is shown in Fig. 4.

```
[demonstration list]
question: [input of demonstration #1]
answer: [output of demonstration #1]
......
question: [input of demonstration #n]
answer: [output of demonstration #n]
Please answer the following questions based on the
example above: replace [test input] with N/A
answer: probability of outputting specific options
```

Fig. 4. Content-free prompt for probability calibration

5   Conclusion

This paper proposed a an in-context-learning framework for health information extraction. All demonstrations in candidate set are scored first, then combined based on their score and length, finally filled into prompt template in a specific order. We traverse candidate combinations and determine eventual methods based on performance on the validation set. Our method achieved 40.27 points in final test set and achieved the first place among five teams, demonstrating the effectiveness of the retrieval paradigm.

Our proposed paradigm could be easily generalized in other LLM-based natural language processing tasks with validation sets and has a good robustness. In the future, we hope to explore how to get the optimal retrieval strategy when migrating the paradigm to unseen tasks for the sake of time and cost reduction.

References

1. Wan, Z., et al.: GPT-RE: in-context learning for relation extraction using large language models. CoRR, abs/2305.02105 (2023)
2. Zhu, W., Wang, X., Zheng, H., Chen, M., Tang, B.: PromptCBLUE: a Chinese prompt tuning benchmark for the medical domain (2023)
3. Brown, T.B., et al.: Language models are few-shot learners. In: Conference on Neural Information Processing Systems, pp. 1877–1901 (2020)
4. Chowdhery, A., et al.: Palm: scaling language modeling with pathways. ICLR 2023 (2022)
5. Taylor, R., et al.: Galactica: a large language model for science. Neural Inf. Process. Syst. (2022)
6. Touvron, H., et al.: Llama 2: open foundation and fine-tuned chat models (2023)
7. Wei, J., et al.: Finetuned language models are zero-shot learners. abs/2109.01652 (2022)

8. Ouyang, L., et al.: Training language models to follow instructions with human feedback (2022)

9. Zhao, W.X., et al.: A survey of large language models. Computing Research Repository, abs/2303.18223 (2023)

10. Dai, D., Sun, Y., Dong, L., Hao, Y., Sui, Z., Wei, F.: Why can GPT learn in-context? Language models secretly perform gradient descent as meta-optimizers. Find. Assoc. Comput. Linguist. ACL **2023**, 4005–4019 (2022)

11. Lin, Y., Ji, H., Huang, F., Wu, L.: A joint neural model for information extraction with global features (2020). 2020.acl-main:7999–8009

12. Wei, X., et al.: Zero-shot information extraction via chatting with chatgpt (2023)

13. Li, B., et al.: Evaluating chatgpt's information extraction capabilities: sn assessment of performance, explainability, calibration, and faithfulness. abs/2304.11633 (2023)

14. Ji, B.: Vicunaner: zero/few-shot named entity recognition using vicuna. arXiv preprint arXiv:2305.03253 (2023)

15. Wadhwa, S., Amir, S., Wallace, B.C.: Revisiting relation extraction in the era of large language models. abs/2305.05003:15566–15589 (2023)

16. Radford, A., Wu, J., Child, R., Luan, D., Amodei, D., Sutskever, I.: Language models are unsupervised multitask learners (2019)

17. Zhang, B., Sennrich, R.: Root mean square layer normalization. Adv. Neural. Inf. Process. Syst. **32**, 12360–12371 (2019)

18. Shazeer, N.: GLU variants improve transformer (2020)

19. Su, J., Ahmed, M., Lu, Y., Pan, S., Bo, W., Liu, Y.: Roformer: enhanced transformer with rotary position embedding. semanticscholar, abs/2104.09864 (2022)

20. Zhang, Z., et al.: Auto-instruct: automatic instruction generation and ranking for black-box language models (2023)

21. Gao, S., Wen, X.C., Gao, C., Wang, W., Zhang, H., Lyu, M.R.: What makes good in-context demonstrations for code intelligence tasks with LLMs? ASE, abs/2304.07575 (2023)

22. Trotman, A., Puurula, A., Burgess, B.: Improvements to BM25 and language models examined. In: Proceedings of the 19th Australasian Document Computing Symposium, pp. 58–65 (2014)

23. Xu, M.: text2vec: a tool for text to vector (2023)

24. Zhao, Z., Wallace, E., Feng, S., Klein, D., Singh, S.: Calibrate before use: improving few-shot performance of language models. In: International Conference on Machine Learning, pp. 12697–12706 (2021)

ECNU-LLM@CHIP-PromptCBLUE: Prompt Optimization and In-Context Learning for Chinese Medical Tasks

Huanran Zheng, Ming Guan[✉], Yihan Mei, Yanjun Li, and Yuanbin Wu

East China Normal University, Shanghai, China
{hrzheng,51265901114,51265901097,51265901098}@stu.ecnu.edu.cn,
ybwu@cs.ecnu.edu.cn

Abstract. Our team, ECNU-LLM, presents a method of in-context learning for enhancing the performance of large language models without fine-tuning in the 9th China Health Information Processing Conference (CHIP 2023) Open Shared Task PromptCBLUE-v2 evaluation task (http://www.cips-chip.org.cn/2023/eval1). Our method contains the following steps: (1) Initially, we employ text retrieval models to select the top demonstrations from the training set based on the similarity scores. (2) Furthermore, we handle different tasks separately by adding prompts according to their task types. (3) For certain tasks, the chain-of-thought approach is employed to further improve performance. (4) Finally, we improve the post-processing scripts provided by the task organizers, enabling more efficient extraction of information from large model language outputs. Using this approach, we utilize Baichuan-13B-Chat to directly generate predictions on the test set, achieving a score of 39.25 in the CHIP2023-PromptCBLUE-no fine-tuning track.

Keywords: LLM · PromptCBLUE · In-context Learning · Chain-of-Thought

1 Introduction

Increasingly large pre-trained models [1–6] built upon the Transformer architecture [7–9] have been emerging and achieving the state-of-the-art (SOTA) results on a variety of downstream tasks [10–22]. However, these models require fine-tuning for downstream task adaptations. With the continuous releases of large language models (LLMs) represented by ChatGPT and GPT-4[1], the LLM revolution has sparked a new wave of research in the field of Natural Language Processing (NLP) [23–28], in-context learning. LLMs demonstrate proficiency in various NLP tasks and have robust zero-shot learning capabilities and the ability to learn and infer according to the in-context information [29–31].

---

[1] https://chat.openai.com/.

H. Xu et al. (Eds.): CHIP 2023, CCIS 2080, pp. 60–72, 2024.
https://doi.org/10.1007/978-981-97-1717-0_5

The PromptCBLUE-v2 [32,33] benchmark, as a secondary development of the CBLUE benchmark, has transformed 18 different medical scenario NLP tasks into prompt-based language generation tasks. This benchmark aims to establish a unified form of NLP tasks within the Chinese medical NLP community. These tasks include information extraction, medical concept normalization, medical text classification, medical dialogue understanding and generation, etc., forming the first Chinese medical scenario LLM evaluation benchmark.

In the track that allows prediction using only specified open-source large language model backbones without fine-tuning, we utilize Baichuan-13B-Chat as the base model for the PromptCBLUE-v2 evaluation tasks in the CHIP background. We introduce prompt optimization strategies, leverage demonstrations selection from the training set for in-context learning to enhance the model's performance, and finally enhance the accuracy of the evaluation results through post-processing strategies. In the end, our approach achieved a score of 39.25 on the final leaderboard, ranking second and highlighting its significant effectiveness.

Specifically, the framework of prompt optimization and in-context learning proposed in this paper consists of three main parts:

1. To enable LLM to generate more accurate responses to tasks with strong causality, we use the Chain-of-Thought (CoT) method [34] to optimize prompts in some specific tasks.
2. We employ an in-context learning strategy to guide LLM in its generation process. During in-context learning, we use the auxiliary sentence representation model bge-base-zh-v1.5 [35] to find the top n samples from the training set that are most similar to the current query as demonstrations to guide LLM's generation process. Notably, the number of the selected demonstrations varies across different tasks, and an excessive number of demonstrations does not necessarily lead to more accurate LLM outputs. Therefore, we conduct comprehensive hyperparameter experiments to decide the number of instances for each task.
3. To improve the accuracy of LLM's inference in the final submission, we propose a post-processing strategy. Since the evaluation standards for the majority of tasks rely primarily on the F1-score, the main function of the post-processing strategy is to standardize generated characters, reduce invalid outputs, and ignore erroneous outputs, ultimately making the final submission results more accurate.

2   Related Work

In this section, we introduce some work related to the methods in this paper, including prompt engineering, in-context learning, and semantic retrieval.

2.1   Prompt Engineering

Some researchers have found that using prompt can significantly improve the performance of pre-trained language models in downstream applications [36].

Therefore, how to effectively construct prompt has become a popular research direction. Since manually constructing prompts is too labor-intensive, some researchers have proposed methods for automatically designing prompts. For example, Shin et al. [37] proposed a discrete word space search algorithm based on downstream application training data. Although this technology is better than manual prompt design, the expressive ability of discrete prompts is weak and the improvement for downstream tasks is small. Therefore, some researchers proposed a prompt tuning [38] method to optimize continuous prompt vectors through gradient backpropagation. This type of method can achieve good performance, but since parameter fine-tuning is prohibited in this track, we adopted the approach of manually designing prompts.

2.2 In-Context Learning

In-context learning (ICL) is a learning paradigm that leverages LLMs to perform complex tasks by providing a few relevant demonstrations or instructions in the context. ICL has been applied to various natural language processing (NLP) tasks, such as text classification, question answering, text generation, and so on. For example, Brown et al. [36] showed that GPT-3 can achieve competitive results on several NLP benchmarks by using ICL with a few demonstrations. Zhou et al. [39] proposed an automatic prompt engineering method to generate and select task instructions for ICL. Wei et al. [34] introduced a Chain-of-Thoughts (CoT) prompting method to enhance the inference ability of LLMs by adding intermediate steps between inputs and outputs of demonstrations.

The selection of examples affects the performance of in-context learning [30]. Margatina et al. [40] explored what kind of demonstrations can best help the model perform in-context learning. Specifically, they compared three demonstration construction methods: diversity-based, uncertainty-based, and similarity-based. Through experiments, they found that demonstrations with high semantic similarity to the input performed best. Therefore, in this paper, we adopt a semantic retrieval model to retrieve samples with high semantic similarity to the input as demonstrations.

2.3 Semantic Retrieval

Semantic retrieval is a vector-based retrieval technology that returns the most relevant results based on the intent and context of the search query, rather than just keyword matching. The advantage of semantic retrieval is that it can improve the accuracy and relevance of search results, as well as handle some complex natural language queries, such as paraphrasing, error correction, transformation and generalization. The core of semantic retrieval is how to convert text into vectors and how to calculate the similarity or distance between vectors. Semantic retrieval has been applied to a variety of natural language processing tasks, such as document retrieval, question answering systems, text summarization, etc. For example, Guu et al. [41] proposed a method for semantic retrieval using a LLM, called REALM, which can dynamically update the vector representation of a document during the retrieval process. Li et al. [42] proposed a method using contrastive learning, called ColBERT, which can use fine-grained vector representation during retrieval. Zhang et al. [43] proposed a method using knowledge graphs, called KEPLER, which can use structured knowledge to enhance the vector representation of text, thereby improving the semantic relevance of retrieval. Recently, Xiao et al. [35] introduced a package of resources that significantly advance the field of general Chinese embeddings, and the models they provide perform very well on the MTEB benchmark [44]. Therefore, we adopt bge-base-zh-v1.5 as our semantic embedding model.

3   Method

PromptCBLUE-v2 benchmark has conducted secondary development on the CBLUE benchmark and transformed 18 different NLP tasks in the medical domain into prompt-based language generation tasks. The competition also introduced an untuned track, which requires participants to directly predict the test set using a specified large open source model backbone. The challenge lies in the restriction that no fine-tuning of the open-source large model is allowed, and no additional parameters can be added to the large model. Therefore, one possible approach is to use in-context learning to improve the performance of given large language models.

Our approach proposes three optimization methods to enhance the performance of large language models. Firstly, we utilize the CoT technique to modify the prompts for tasks with strong causal relationships. Secondly, we employ a sentence embedding model to assist the model in selecting demonstrations from the training set for each different test sample. Finally, we modify the post-processing procedure to extract key information from the generated results of the large model.

3.1   Chain of Thought

CoT prompting is proven to be effective in boosting the reasoning capabilities of LLMs under the zero-shot setting and few-shot ICL setting [34]. [45,46] also demonstrate that CoT is beneficial for LLM fine-tuning on complex information extraction tasks. We now provide reasoning paths on how to derive specific answers for tasks with strong causal relationships such as KUAKE-QQR and CMedCasual. This helps the model better capture step-by-step thinking processes. For example, the KUAKE-QQR task involves determining the semantic relationship between two medical queries.

As shown in Fig. 1, in the original input, the model input includes a description of the task type, where Example 1 and Example n are valuable demonstrations selected from the training data. Example n+1 is the true query, and the model output is to choose one of the following four semantic relationships to answer: ["completely consistent", "the latter is a semantic subset of the former",

"the latter is a semantic superset of the former", "no semantic association"].
However, the model doesn't understand the reasons behind these four semantic
relationships, leading to biased results. To address this issue, we provide specific
reasoning paths to the model, ultimately achieving correct results and enhancing
the model's performance.

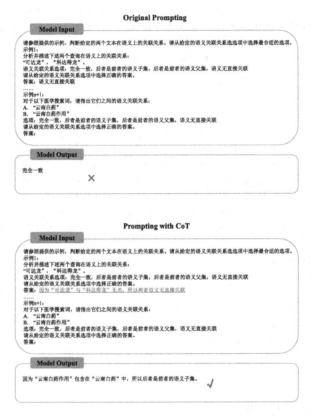

Fig. 1. An example of constructing chain-of-thought prompts in the KUAKE-QQR
task. Compared with the original prompt, chain-of-thought prompt adds the corresponding reasoning path before outputting the label for each demonstrations.

3.2 BGE

Randomly selecting training data as demonstrations can improve model performance, but this method is not stable and may lead to a decrease in performance.
To address this issue, we adopt a method based on retrieving documents related
to the test data, which has significantly improved the model's performance.

We introduce the BGE (Graph-based Text Embedding) method [35]. BGE
maps text data to a low-dimensional space for retrieval and similarity calculation.
It focuses on the semantic structure of text data and can provide better semantic

relevance. In this paper, we use the bge-base-zhv1.5 model to compute output vectors for all data in the training set for retrieval.

As shown in Fig. 2, we calculate the cosine similarity between the representation vector of the current input sentence and the retrieval vectors of the training set data, selecting the top-n data with the highest similarity as demonstrations. Then, the training data is arranged as demonstrations 1-n in descending order of similarity scores. The current input is considered as demonstrations n+1. The number of demonstrations depends on the specific task, as detailed in the experiment section.

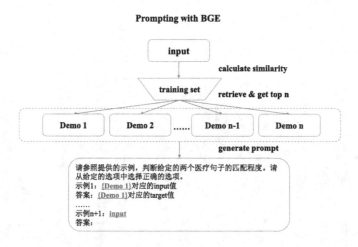

Fig. 2. A BGE flow chart in the KUAKE-QTR task.

3.3   Post-processing

In the experiment, we discover that the post-processing program provided by the task organizers is not effectively extracting the correct answers from the outputs generated by large language models. Therefore, it is necessary to modify the post-processing program. The major modifications include:

- Unify the format of punctuation marks.
- Use heuristic rules to delete obviously wrong answers.
- For classification tasks, if the result generated by the model is not in the label list, a label is randomly sampled as the final answer.

4   Experiments

4.1   Datasets and Evaluation Metrics

PromptCBLUE-v2 [32] adds prompts to the previous Chinese medical datasets of various tasks and unifies them into a form that LLM can process. These dataset consists 18 subtasks and can be divided into the five groups: Medical information extraction (CMeEE-V2, CMeIE-V2, CHIP-CDEE, CHIP-CDN, IMCS-V2-NER, Text2DT [46,47], CMedCausal), Medical text classification (CHIP-CTC, KUAKE-QIC, IMCS-V2-DAC), Medical natural language inference tasks (CHIP-STS, KUAKE-QQR, KUAKE-IR, KUAKE-QTR), Symptom status understanding for medical dialogues (IMCS-V2-SR, CHIP-MDCFNPC) and Medical content generation (IMCS-V2-MRG, MedDG). The number of each subtask in the training set is shown in Fig. 3.

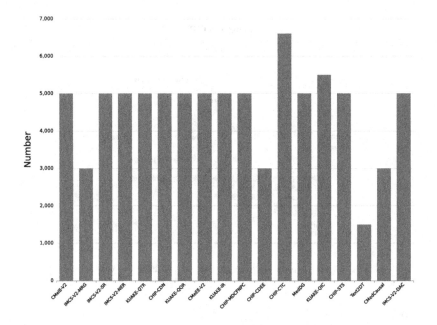

Fig. 3. Number of each subtask in training set.

The evaluation metrics for different subtasks are different, including:

1. Micro-F1 metric for CMeEE-V2, CMeIE-V2, CHIP-CDN, CHIP-CDEE, IMCS-V2-NER, CHIP-MDCFNPC, IMCS-V2-SR, CHIP-STS, KUAKE-IR, KUAKE-QQR, KUAKE-QTR, CMedCausal.
2. Macro-F1 metric for IMCS-V2-DAC, CHIP-CTC, KUAKE-QIC.
3. TreeLenvRatio metric for Text2DT.
4. Rouge metric for MedDG, IMCS-V2-MRG.

The final score is the average of the scores on 18 subtasks.

4.2   Experimental Setup

We adopt Baichuan-13B-Chat[2] as our base model. We use bge-base-zh-v1.5 [35] as our semantic retrieval model to retrieve relevant demonstrations in the training set. During inference, we use beam search for decoding and set the beam to 4. In order to determine the number of demonstrations required for different subtasks, we randomly sampled the validation set and conducted hyperparameter experiments on the sampled validation set. The original validation set contains a total of 7656 data, the validation set we sampled contains 1145 data, and the amount of data contained in each subtask is between 50–100.

Table 1. In-context learning performance of different number of demonstrations in our sampled validation set.

Subtasks	Demonstrations Num							
	0	1	2	3	4	5	6	7
CMeEE-V2	–	31.9	32.3	33.1	33.2	34.2	**34.6**	34.3
CMeIE-V2	–	–	7.6	8.3	8.4	8.6	**9.3**	8.9
CHIP-CDN	–	–	31.7	32.5	36.4	43.5	**46.5**	35.6
CHIP-CDEE	–	–	–	21.3	21.7	22.0	23.7	**26.8**
IMCS-V2-NER	–	–	–	44.0	45.1	46.6	52.1	**52.3**
CHIP-MDCFNPC	–	–	–	37.7	38.5	38.9	**42.5**	38.3
IMCS-V2-SR	–	16.3	24.7	36.9	36.7	37.8	**41.4**	37.9
CHIP-STS	–	–	–	60.5	61.7	**64.2**	63.8	63.7
KUAKE-IR	–	70.1	72.5	**73.7**	72.2	–	–	–
KUAKE-QQR	–	–	32.2	32.3	**37.4**	34.3	33.7	–
KUAKE-QTR	–	–	40.2	40.3	**46.6**	45.0	37.0	–
CMedCausal	–	6.1	6.3	**6.5**	6.4	5.9	–	–
IMCS-V2-DAC	**19.9**	18.3	17.7	16.0	14.6	–	–	–
CHIP-CTC	–	38.1	46.3	47.4	48.1	55.8	**56.1**	47.7
KUAKE-QIC	–	35.1	37.9	40.3	46.9	56.6	**57.5**	46.9
Text2DT	–	48.1	**51.1**	47.7	47.6	–	–	–
MedDG	**14.9**	13.6	13.7	13.1	–	–	–	–
IMCS-V2-MRG	–	31.2	32.7	**33.6**	32.6	32.5	–	–

4.3   Analysis

Effect of Number of Demonstrations The number of demonstrations is a key factor affecting in-context learning. Therefore, we conducted experiments on our sampled validation set to determine the appropriate number of demonstrations for each subtask. The experimental results are shown in Table 1. As we can

---

[2] https://huggingface.co/baichuan-inc/Baichuan-13B-Chat.

see, providing more demonstrations is not always better. Different tasks have different requirements for the number of demonstrations, and some tasks even perform better with zero-shot. We select the number of demonstrations with the best performance in each subtask as the hyperparameters in the final test.

Effect of Chain of Thought As the size of the model increases, some researchers have found that LLM has powerful reasoning capabilities that small models do not have. Therefore, the CoT Prompting method [34] is proposed, which can guide LLM to think deeply, thus improving the accuracy of the final answer. Therefore, we selected two subtasks suitable for using the Chain of Thought Prompting method, selected several demonstrations from the training set, and manually wrote the reasoning process to compare with ordinary retrieved demonstrations. As shown in Table 2, on these two subtasks, using CoT performed better than retrieving demonstrations, so in the final testing stage, we used CoT to construct demonstrations on these two subtasks.

Table 2. Comparison of retrieved demonstrations and Chain of Thought prompting methods on KUAKE-QQR and CMedCausal subtasks.

Method	KUAKE-QQR	CMedCausal
Retrieved Demonstrations	37.4	6.5
Chain of Thought Prompting	45.1	7.3

4.4 Experiments Result

Table 3 shows the performance of our method on all subtasks in the test set. As we can see, our method performs differently on different tasks, and we can achieve higher scores on KUAKE-IR and CHIP-STS tasks. On the CMeIE-V2 and CMedCausal tasks, our scores were lower. We believe this is because these two tasks are complex and too difficult for Baichuan-13B-Chat without fine-tuning. Finally, our overall score on the test set was **39.25**.

Table 3. Performance on different subtasks in the test set. The final average overall score was **39.25**.

CHIP-MDCFNPC	CMeIE-V2	CMedCausal	CHIP-CDEE	IMCS-V2-NER	IMCS-V2-SR	CHIP-STS	KUAKE-IR	KUAKE-QQR
39.79	7.95	7.10	26.83	51.53	37.35	64.25	73.58	45.11
CMeEE-V2	KUAKE-QTR	CHIP-CDN	IMCS-V2-DAC	CHIP-CTC	KUAKE-QIC	Text2DT	MedDG	IMCS-V2-MRG
35.05	40.67	44.56	18.92	56.06	57.61	51.85	14.48	33.79

5   Conclusion

This paper proposes a novel approach for the PromptCBLUE benchmark using Baichuan-13B-Chat as the base model. Building upon this foundation, we enhance the performance of the large language model through three optimization methods without fine-tuning the base model. Firstly, for tasks with strong causality, we utilize chain of thought method to guide the large language model in forming a step-by-step thinking process. Secondly, we use in-context learning methods and employ additional sentence representation models to help select valuable demonstrations. Thirdly, we modify the post-processing procedure to obtain greater accuracy in final submission. Ultimately, our approach achieved a score of 39.25 in the final leaderboard of the race track.

References

1. Han, X., et al.: Pre-trained models: past, present and future. ArXiv, abs/2106.07139 (2021)
2. Devlin, J., Chang, M. W., Lee, K., Toutanova, K.: BERT: pre-training of deep bidirectional transformers for language understanding. In: Proceedings of the 2019 Conference of the North American Chapter of the Association for Computational Linguistics: Human Language Technologies, Volume 1 (Long and Short Papers), pp. 4171–4186, Minneapolis, Minnesota, June 2019. Association for Computational Linguistics (2019)
3. Peters, M.E., et al.: Deep contextualized word representations. In: North American Chapter of the Association for Computational Linguistics (2018)
4. Liu, Y., et al.: Roberta: a robustly optimized bert pretraining approach. arXiv preprint arXiv:1907.11692 (2019)
5. Radford, A., Narasimhan, K.: Improving language understanding by generative pre-training (2018)
6. Raffel, C., et al.: Exploring the limits of transfer learning with a unified text-to-text transformer. ArXiv, abs/1910.10683 (2019)
7. Vaswani, A., et al.: Attention is all you need. ArXiv, abs/1706.03762 (2017)
8. Zhu, W., Wang, X., Ni, Y., Xie, G.: AutoTrans: automating transformer design via reinforced architecture search. In: Wang, L., Feng, Y., Hong, Yu., He, R. (eds.) NLPCC 2021. LNCS (LNAI), vol. 13028, pp. 169–182. Springer, Cham (2021). https://doi.org/10.1007/978-3-030-88480-2_14
9. Zhu, W.: AutoNLU: architecture search for sentence and cross-sentence attention modeling with re-designed search space. In: Wang, L., Feng, Y., Hong, Yu., He, R. (eds.) NLPCC 2021. LNCS (LNAI), vol. 13028, pp. 155–168. Springer, Cham (2021). https://doi.org/10.1007/978-3-030-88480-2_13
10. Gao, X., Zhu, W., Gao, J., Yin, C.: F-PABEE: flexible-patience-based early exiting for single-label and multi-label text classification tasks. In: ICASSP 2023–2023 IEEE International Conference on Acoustics, Speech and Signal Processing (ICASSP), pp. 1–5. IEEE (2023)
11. Zhang, Y., Gao, X., Zhu, W., Wang, X.: Fastner: speeding up inferences for named entity recognition tasks. In: International Conference on Advanced Data Mining and Applications (2023)
12. Zhang, X., Tan, M., Zhang, J., Zhu, W.: NAG-NER: a unified non-autoregressive generation framework for various NER tasks. In: Annual Meeting of the Association for Computational Linguistics (2023)
13. Zheng, H., Zhu, W., Wang, P., Wang, X.: Candidate soups: fusing candidate results improves translation quality for non-autoregressive translation. ArXiv, abs/2301.11503 (2023)

14. Wang, X., et al.: Multi-task entity linking with supervision from a taxonomy. Knowl. Inf. Syst. **65**, 4335–4358 (2023)

15. Zhu, W., Wang, P., Wang, X., Ni, Y., Xie, G.: ACF: aligned contrastive finetuning for language and vision tasks. In: ICASSP 2023–2023 IEEE International Conference on Acoustics, Speech and Signal Processing (ICASSP), pp. 1–5 (2023)

16. Li, X., et al.: Pingan smart health and SJTU at COIN - shared task: utilizing pretrained language models and common-sense knowledge in machine reading tasks. In: Proceedings of the First Workshop on Commonsense Inference in Natural Language Processing, pp. 93–98, Hong Kong, China, November 2019. Association for Computational Linguistics (2019)

17. Zhu, W.: AutoRC: improving BERT based relation classification models via architecture search. In: Proceedings of the 59th Annual Meeting of the Association for Computational Linguistics and the 11th International Joint Conference on Natural Language Processing: Student Research Workshop, pp. 33–43, Online, August 2021. Association for Computational Linguistics (2021)

18. Zuo, Y., Zhu, W., Cai, G.G.: Continually detection, rapidly react: unseen rumors detection based on continual prompt-tuning. In: Proceedings of the 29th International Conference on Computational Linguistics, pp. 3029–3041, Gyeongju, Republic of Korea, October 2022. International Committee on Computational Linguistics (2022)

19. Zhang, Z., Zhu, W., Zhang, J., Wang, P., Jin, R., Chung, T.S.: PCEE-BERT: accelerating BERT inference via patient and confident early exiting. In: Findings of the Association for Computational Linguistics: NAACL 2022, pp. 327–338, Seattle, United States, July 2022. Association for Computational Linguistics (2022)

20. Zhu, W., Wang, X., Ni, Y., Xie, G.: GAML-BERT: improving BERT early exiting by gradient aligned mutual learning. In: Proceedings of the 2021 Conference on Empirical Methods in Natural Language Processing, pp. 3033–3044, Online and Punta Cana, Dominican Republic, November 2021. Association for Computational Linguistics (2021)

21. Guo, Z., Ni, Y., Wang, K., Zhu, W., Xie, G.: Global attention decoder for Chinese spelling error correction. In: Findings of the Association for Computational Linguistics: ACL-IJCNLP 2021, pp. 1419–1428, Online, August 2021. Association for Computational Linguistics (2021)

22. Zhu, W., et al.: paht_nlp @ MEDIQA 2021: multi-grained query focused multi-answer summarization. In: Proceedings of the 20th Workshop on Biomedical Language Processing, pp. 96–102, Online, June 2021. Association for Computational Linguistics (2021)

23. Cui, G., et al.: Ultrafeedback: boosting language models with high-quality feedback. ArXiv, abs/2310.01377 (2023)

24. Zhu, W., Tan, M.: SPT: learning to selectively insert prompts for better prompt tuning. In: Bouamor, H., Pino, J., Bali, K. (eds.), Proceedings of the 2023 Conference on Empirical Methods in Natural Language Processing, pp. 11862–11878, Singapore, December 2023. Association for Computational Linguistics (2023)

25. Zhang, Y., Wang, P., Tan, M., Zhu, W.: Learned adapters are better than manually designed adapters. In: Annual Meeting of the Association for Computational Linguistics (2023)

26. Sun, T., et al.: A simple hash-based early exiting approach for language understanding and generation. In: Findings of the Association for Computational Linguistics: ACL 2022, pp. 2409–2421, Dublin, Ireland, May 2022. Association for Computational Linguistics (2022)

27. Zuo, Y., Zhu, W., Cai, G.G.: Continually detection, rapidly react: unseen rumors detection based on continual prompt-tuning. In: COLING (2022)
28. Zhang, J., Tan, M., Dai, P., Zhu, W.: LECO: improving early exiting via learned exits and comparison-based exiting mechanism. In: Annual Meeting of the Association for Computational Linguistics (2023)
29. Liu, J., Shen, D., Zhang, Y., Dolan, B., Carin, L., Chen, W.: What makes good in-context examples for GPT-3? In: Workshop on Knowledge Extraction and Integration for Deep Learning Architectures, Deep Learning Inside Out (2021)
30. Li, X., et al.: Unified demonstration retriever for in-context learning. ArXiv, abs/2305.04320 (2023)
31. Zhu, W., Wang, P., Ni, Y., Xie, G., Wang, X.: BADGE: speeding up BERT inference after deployment via block-wise bypasses and divergence-based early exiting. In: Annual Meeting of the Association for Computational Linguistics (2023)
32. Zhu, W., Wang, X., Zheng, H., Chen, M., Tang, B.: PromptCBLUE: a Chinese prompt tuning benchmark for the medical domain. ArXiv, abs/2310.14151 (2023)
33. Zhu, W., Wang, X., Chen, M., Tang, B.: Overview of the PromptCBLUE shared task in CHIP2023 (2023)
34. Wei, J., et al.: Chain of thought prompting elicits reasoning in large language models. ArXiv, abs/2201.11903 (2022)
35. Xiao, S., Liu, Z., Zhang, P., Muennighof, N.: C-PACK: packaged resources to advance general Chinese embedding (2023)
36. Brown, T., et al.: Language models are few-shot learners. Adv. Neural Inf. Process. Syst. **33**, 1877–1901 (2020)
37. Shin, T., Razeghi, Y., Logan IV, R.L., Wallace, E., Singh, S.: AutoPrompt: eliciting knowledge from language models with automatically generated prompts. In: Webber, B., Cohn, T., He, Y., Liu, Y. (eds.), Proceedings of the 2020 Conference on Empirical Methods in Natural Language Processing (EMNLP), pp. 4222–4235, Online, November 2020. Association for Computational Linguistics (2020)
38. Lester, B., Al-Rfou, R., Constant, N.: The power of scale for parameter-efficient prompt tuning. In: Conference on Empirical Methods in Natural Language Processing (2021)
39. Shin, T., Razeghi, Y., Logan IV, R.L., Wallace, E., Singh, S.: Autoprompt: eliciting knowledge from language models with automatically generated prompts. arXiv preprint arXiv:2010.15980 (2020)
40. Margatina, K., Schick, T., Aletras, N., Dwivedi-Yu, J.: Active learning principles for in-context learning with large language models. ArXiv, abs/2305.14264 (2023)
41. Guu, K., Lee, K., Tung, Z., Pasupat, P., Chang, M.: Retrieval augmented language model pre-training. In: International Conference on Machine Learning, pp. 3929–3938. PMLR (2020)
42. Khattab, O., Zaharia, M.: ColBERT: efficient and effective passage search via contextualized late interaction over BERT (2020)
43. Wang, X., et al.: KEPLER: a unified model for knowledge embedding and pre-trained language representation. Trans. Assoc. Comput. Linguist. **9**, 176–194 (2021)
44. Muennighoff, N., Tazi, N., Magne, L., Reimers, N.: MTEB: massive text embedding benchmark. In: Conference of the European Chapter of the Association for Computational Linguistics (2022)
45. Zhu, W., Wang, X., Zheng, H., Chen, M., Tang, B.: PromptCBLUE: a Chinese prompt tuning benchmark for the medical domain, October 2023. arXiv e-prints, page arXiv:2310.14151

46. Zhu, W., et al.: Text2MDT: extracting medical decision trees from medical texts, January 2024. arXiv e-prints, page arXiv:2401.02034
47. Zhu, W., et al.: Extracting decision trees from medical texts: an overview of the Text2DT track in CHIP2022. In: Tang, B., et al. (eds.) Health Information Processing. Evaluation Track Papers. CHIP 2022. CCIS, vol. 1773, pp. 89–102. Springer, Singapore (2023). https://doi.org/10.1007/978-981-99-4826-0_9

Similarity-Based Prompt Construction for Large Language Model in Medical Tasks

Gaofei Liu[1], Meiqi Pan[1], Zhiyuan Ma[1,2(✉)], Miaomiao Gu[1], Ling Yang[1], and Jiwei Qin[1]

[1] Institute of Machine Intelligence, University of Shanghai for Science and Technology, Shanghai, China
{223332595,222302289,233352471,232322306, 213332821}@st.usst.edu.cn, yuliar3514@usst.edu.cn
[2] State Key Laboratory for Novel Software Technology, Nanjing University, Nanjing, China

Abstract. Large Language Model (LLM) has sparked a new trend in Natural Language Processing (NLP), and an increasing number of researches have recognized the potential of using LLM to unify diverse NLP tasks into a text generative manner. In order to explore the potential of LLM for In-Context Learning in Chinese Medical field, the 9th China Health Information Processing Conference (CHIP 2023) has released a non-tuning LLM evaluation task called PromptCBLUE-v2. In this paper, we proposed a similarity-based prompt construction method which ranked the third place in the final list. It follows the framework of demonstration-based prompt template and uses sentence-level similarity to select representative sentences for better demonstration. To avoid unformatted output, we designed a two-round conversation method. Additionally, we incorporated similarity model to evaluate answer similarity to convert unformatted output to desired target answer. The evaluations on 18 NLP tasks have proved the generalization and effectiveness of our method.

Keywords: Large Language Model · CHIP 2023 · similarity-based · In-Context Learning

1 Introduction

With the popularization of ChatGPT, Large Language Model (LLM) has motivated an increasing trend in both industry and academic. An increasing number of researches are transforming conventional NLP tasks into prompt-based text generation tasks [1–5]. Following the trend, the PromptCBLUE-v2 evaluation benchmark introduced in the CHIP2023 evaluation task converts 18 different Chinese medical domain datasets containing 8 traditional tasks into a unified prompt-based text generation task. It is a secondary development based on the CBLUE [6] evaluation benchmark. At the same time, PromptCBLUE-v2 benchmark has undergone a more comprehensive upgrade compared to the PromptCBLUE [7] benchmark. Two new datasets, Text2DT [8] and CMedCausal, have been added to the PromptCBLUE-v2 benchmark. The number of prompt templates

H. Xu et al. (Eds.): CHIP 2023, CCIS 2080, pp. 73–83, 2024.
https://doi.org/10.1007/978-981-97-1717-0_6

provided by the organizers has also increased from 94 in PromptCBLUE to over 450. It poses a greater challenge for LLMs and increases the demand for robustness. In order to investigate different techniques in the field of LLMs, this evaluation task provides two tracks: efficient fine-tuning of LLM parameters and non-tuning [9].

The purpose of the non-tuning track in the PromptCBLUE-v2 is to assess the potential of LLM in In-Context Learning (ICL) [10]. Through the adoption of ICL, the LLM can predict test samples based on a small number of training samples as demonstrations without tuning any parameters. Therefore, in this article, we follow the paradigm by selecting demonstrations from training set. Recent studies indicate that ICL is highly sensitive to input prompts [11–14]. Based on their works, we believe that there are two key problems. Firstly, how to select appropriate demonstrations for each test sample to construct high-quality inputs. Secondly, how to standardize the output format of LLM. To solve them, we proposed a Similarity-based Prompt Construction method called Sim-PC. Meanwhile, we explored the memory capabilities of the LLM to design a two-round conversation method, which enables the LLM to use the knowledge from previous conversation to formatting the output. In the end, we achieved a commendable score in the evaluation track, which also validated the effectiveness of our approach.

The main contributions are summarized as follows:

- To select appropriate demonstrations, we proposed a similarity-based prompt construction method specifically for Chinese medical texts.
- We designed a two-round conversation approach to format the output.
- Our proposed method achieved commendable results in the non-tuning track of the PromptCBLUE-v2 evaluation benchmark.

2 Preliminaries

With the prevalence of LLMs in both academic and industrial domains, an increasing amount of researches are exploring the potential of LLMs [1–3], leading to the proposal of new paradigms for NLP tasks. A new paradigm called In-Context Learning (ICL) [10] uses input-label pairs as demonstrations to guide LLMs to directly predict test samples without updating any parameters, and has achieved remarkable performance [15, 16]. ICL has garnered widespread attention, with a considerable amount of research effort dedicated to studying this task. Recent researches [11–14] have shown that ICL is highly sensitive to input prompts, and randomly selecting demonstrations may have a negative impact on the performance. The phenomenon further motivated them to study how the selection and order of demonstrations can influence prediction. There have been efforts dedicated to studying how to select appropriate examples to improve prediction accuracy [12, 17, 18]. Li et al. [19] proposed UDR, a single model for demonstration retrieval across a wide range of tasks, which focuses on learning various tasks' demonstration retrieval in a unified form. Min et al. [20] researched the impact of label noise on ICL and also proposed some methods to improve the accuracy of ICL. In addition, there are many studies attempting to explore how the transformer architecture achieves the ability for ICL [21–23]. They explore the internal mechanisms through which transformers achieve the ability for ICL by modeling ICL task using various classical machine learning algorithms.

3   In-Context Learning with Similarity-Based Prompt Construction

The PromptCBLUE-v2 benchmark includes 18 datasets, each of which belonging to 8 different NLP tasks, and exhibits extremely high data complexity. In order to obtain a unified framework for NLP tasks through the use of LLM, the current researches focus on the demonstration-based ICL paradigm. In this paper, we have followed the trend and constructed a demonstration-based framework. Different from other prompt-based methods which rely on manually constructed or model-generated template, our framework uses ground truth samples as demonstrations. As mentioned in previous section, we consider that there are two key issues for the framework. One is how to select suitable examples as demonstrations, and the other is how to format the answers generated by the LLM. In this paper, we used similarity-based model for sentence level to choose most related samples in the training set and select TOP-K samples as our demonstrations. To format the answers, we designed a two-round conversation approach for LLM to utilize its own knowledge in formatting the output. To align the answer with target label, we further compared the generated text with the list of optional answers by using the same sentence-level similarity model as we did in the demonstration selection. The overall framework of our approach is shown in Fig. 1, and specific details will be introduced in the following subsections.

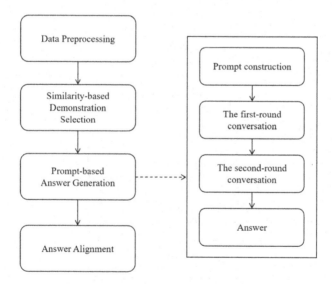

Fig. 1. The overall framework of our approach. On the left are the four main modules of the framework we proposed, each presented from top to bottom. On the right is the expanded explanation of the Prompt-based Answer Generation module.

3.1 Data Preprocessing

For the data used in the task, we performed two main preprocessing steps. Since we wanted to separately input the 18 datasets into the model, our first step involved splitting the mixed data file into 18 separate files based on the dataset. Among the 18 datasets released for this evaluation task, there are over 450 prompt templates included in the inputs. Each input can be directly used as an input for a large model to make predictions. However, the accuracy of these predictions is greatly influenced by the quality of the provided prompt templates. Moreover, a single test text alone may not effectively convey the intended meaning to the large model. Therefore, we will use demonstrations as a way to guide the large model in making predictions for the test samples. In order to calculate text similarity during the subsequent example selection process, our second step involved removing all the 450+ templates provided by the organizers from the data. This resulted in a clean dataset consisting only of pure medical text, which served as a foundation for further operations.

3.2 Similarity-Based Demonstration Selection

Selecting appropriate demonstrations from the training set for guiding the LLM to perform high-quality ICL is crucial for the testing text. In this step, we utilized an open-source Chinese similarity model called RoFormer-Sim[1].

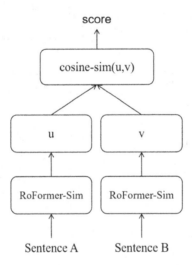

Fig. 2. Similarity score calculation method. For the sentences A and B that require similarity calculation, firstly, the RoFormer-Sim model is used to convert the two sentences into sentence vectors u and v, and then the co-sine similarity of the sentence vectors u and v is calculated to obtain the similarity score between sentence A and sentence B.

---

[1] RoFormer-Sim: https://github.com/ZhuiyiTechnology/roformer-sim.

This model is an upgraded version of SimBERT. Compared with SimBERT, RoFormer-Sim uses more training data and expands to general sentence patterns, which can better meet the complexity of the evaluation task data. RoFormer-Sim is essentially a similarity sentence augmentation model, and calculating the similarity between two sentences as a retrieval model is just one of its auxiliary functions. However, its retrieval performance is indeed outstanding. Regarding the retrieval model, it is inspired by the design philosophy of Sentence-BERT [24]. The retrieval performance of Sentence-BERT has been distilled into RoFormer-Sim, significantly improving its retrieval capability. As shown in Fig. 2, RoFormer-Sim, as a retrieval model, first extracts features from sentences A and B. Then, it calculates the similarity score between the two sentence vectors using cosine similarity.

For each dataset, we calculate the similarity between each test sample and all corresponding training samples to obtain the top 2–3 training samples with the highest similarity to the test sample. In order to prevent the interference of the original instruction templates on the similarity model, both the test samples and training samples here are pure medical texts without the original instruction templates removed.

3.3 Prompt-Based Answer Generation

In order to enable the LLM to use its own knowledge to correct formatting issues in the output, we leverage the memory capacity of the LLM by using a two-round conversation approach. For the selection of the open-source LLM in this evaluation task, we conducted simple testing and comparison, and ultimately chose Baichuan-13B-chat. Figure 3 illustrates a complete conversation process.

For prompt construction, we adopt the approach of combining task prompts, demonstrations, and testing samples. Considering that each dataset involves a different task, creating a unified task prompt may not effectively enable the LLM to understand each task. Therefore, we have designed a dedicated task prompt for each dataset individually. For the combination of demonstrations, We combine the prompt marker "示例:" (Demonstrations:) with a list format, where each individual demonstration sample is treated as an element within the list. To enhance the semantic information of the demonstrations and better guide the large-scale model, we did not use stripped-down instruction templates for our demonstrations. Instead, we retrieved the most original training samples based on their ids. This approach allows us to provide more diverse and context-rich demonstrations for the model's training and inference. Additionally, to prevent interference from noise, we have removed all redundant information from the original demonstrations and retained only the "input" and "target" components. For the testing texts, we strive to maintain consistency with the format of the examples as much as possible. Additionally, to avoid confusion with the demonstrations, the testing samples are also equipped with a testing prompt marker "测试:" (Test:). We concatenate these three components using newline characters ("\n") to form the input for the LLM.

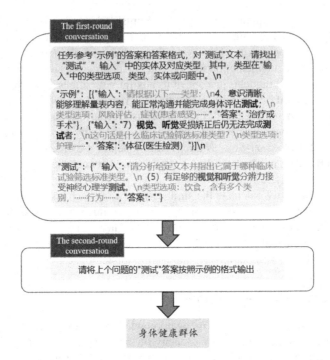

Fig. 3. An example of a complete conversation process. The two boxes contain the inputs for two rounds of conversation. In the first round of conversation, the blue block represents the task prompt for the test sample, the pink block represents the demonstrations selected for that test sample, and the green block represents the test sample. In the second round of conversation, the yellow block represents the input for the second round. After the second round of conversation, LLM will provide a final response. (Color figure online)

For the first round of conversation, we input a well-constructed prompt based on demonstrations to the LLM and let the LLM generate a response. Here we found that the replies from LLM were not fully adhering to the format we specified, so the main purpose of designing the second round of conversation is to allow LLM to use its knowledge to correct and format its own replies. In the end, we only select the final response from LLM as the answer.

3.4 Answer Alignment

For tasks involving answer choices, we found that LLM's responses were generally predicted correctly but with slight differences in expression from the predicted options, which eventually led to prediction errors. Therefore, we performed post-processing on the responses from the LLM to align the answers. Here we once again use the RoFormer-Sim model to calculate the similarity between LLM's response and the answer choices, and select the option with the highest similarity to LLM's response from the list of options as the final answer. An example is shown in Fig. 4.

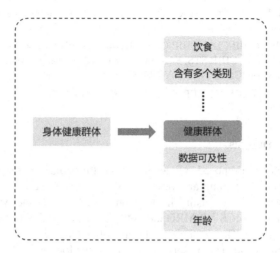

Fig. 4. An example of answer alignment. For classification tasks, the answer generated in the second round of conversation and the answer candidate list are aligned again through similarity calculation. The answer with the highest similarity score (orange block) is selected as the final answer. (Color figure online)

4 Experiments

4.1 Experimental Setup

In this evaluation task, we directly predicted answers for the test set using a demonstrations-guided approach to guide the LLM without tuning any parameters. We selected Baichuan-13B-chat as our final LLM model for all tasks. Additionally, for the selection of demonstrations, we set the quantity to 3. However, for tasks with original sentences that are too long and the LLM has input length limitations, we set the number of demonstrations for these tasks to 2. Detailed information for the settings is provided in Table 1. Each task was processed separately, and for each testing sample, its validation set was discarded, and only data from its corresponding training set was selected. The operating system used was Ubuntu 20.04, running on Python 3.7.16, with transformers 4.30.2 and PyTorch 1.13.1. Hardware support included an NVIDIA RTX A6000 graphics card with 48 GB of memory. For the similarity model RoFormer-Sim, we conducted experiments using the model open-sourced by the original author without making any updates or modifications to the parameters.

Table 1. The parameter settings for the number of demonstrations.

Set to 2	CMeIE-V2, CHIP-CDN, CHIP-CDEE, CHIP-MDCFNPC, IMCS-V2-SR, IMCS-V2-DAC, CHIP-STS, KUAKE-IR, KUAKE-QQR, KUAKE-QTR, MedDG, Text2DT, CMedCausal, IMCS-V2-MRG
Set to 3	CMeEE-V2, IMCS-V2-NER, CHIP-CTC, KUAKE-QIC

4.2 Results and Analysis

With the approach we proposed, we achieved the third place among all participating teams in this task, attaining an average score of 36.8036 across 18 datasets. The Text2DT dataset was evaluated using the decision tree edit rate as the evaluation metric, while the MedDG and IMCS-V2-MRG datasets for the generation tasks were assessed using the Rouge-L score. The remaining datasets utilized the F1 (micro/macro) score as the final evaluation metric. The performance evaluations for each dataset are shown in Table 2. Among them, we obtained the highest scores for the CMeEE-V2 and CHIP-CTC datasets.

Table 2. The performance evaluations for all 18 datasets.

Dataset	Score	Dataset	Score
CMeEE-V2	41.3542	CHIP-STS	59.3379
CMeIE-V2	3.6556	KUAKE-IR	72.8448
CHIP-CDN	42.9112	KUAKE-QIC	59.4799
CHIP-CDEE	19.8755	KUAKE-QQR	44.4595
IMCS-V2-NER	58.2449	KUAKE-QTR	31.3123
CHIP-MDCFNPC	32.1487	MedDG	10.3149
IMCS-V2-SR	29.0664	Text2DT	44.5911
IMCS-V2-DAC	16.1841	CMedCausal	3.0888
CHIP-CTC	65.8387	IMCS-V2-MRG	27.7563

From Table 2, it can be seen that our method performs well in the classification task, but it does not perform as well in the complex relation extraction and generation tasks. Based on this, we believe that handling extremely complex tasks solely relying on ICL without adjusting any parameters of LLM is extremely challenging.

For this evaluation task, we conducted several comparative experiments on selected demonstrations for the CMeEE-V2 dataset. As a Chinese medical named entity recognition (NER) dataset, CMeEE-V2 is a very classic and representative task in all tasks. In addition, the complexity of this task is in the middle of all the data sets of this evaluation task, which is one of the main reasons why we choose it for comparative experiment. For the comparison experiment, at first, we did not choose to use demonstrations, but directly predicted the answers through the task prompts constructed by ourselves on the combination of instruction templates provided by the government as input. In this way, we could only rely on LLM's own knowledge and understanding of Prompt. After our experimental observation, we found that the most fatal problem for this evaluation without demonstrations is that it is difficult to have a fixed output format. In the second experiment, we randomly selected 3 demonstrations for each test sample in the corresponding training set, and then combined them with the task prompts we constructed as inputs for answer prediction. The experiment found that the demonstrations method did have a good effect on the format problem, but the accuracy became the most important problem. In the third experiment, based on the method proposed in this paper, the accuracy and output format problems have been significantly improved, which also proves the effectiveness of our method.

5 Conclusion

In this paper, based on the evaluation task at hand, we are committed to selecting appropriate demonstrations for ICL. At the same time, we attempt to format the output of LLM to ensure the accuracy of the answers. For the selection of demonstrations, we propose a similarity-based demonstration selection method, implementing the open-source text similarity model RoFormer-Sim. For formatting LLM's output, we design a two-round conversation method, using LLM's own knowledge to format the output. Finally, we use the similarity model again to align the answers, ensuring the reliability of the predictions. Through the method we proposed, we have achieved quite promising results in this evaluation task. However, we believe that there is still significant room for improvement in our approach. First, for the medical domain data in this evaluation, using a text similarity model trained on medical data may yield better results. Second, we lack sufficient exploration in the construction of input templates. Constructing suitable input templates for different tasks is crucial for predicting the final answers.

References

1. Shao, W., Hu, Y., Ji, P., Yan, X., Fan, D., Zhang, R.: Prompt-NER: Zero-shot named entity recognition in astronomy literature via large language models. arXiv preprint arXiv:2310. 17892 (2023)
2. Wadhwa, S., Amir, S., Wallace, B.C.: Revisiting relation extraction in the era of large language models. arXiv preprint arXiv:2305.05003 (2023)
3. Chiang, C.H., Lee, H.Y.: Can large language models be an alternative to human evaluations? arXiv preprint arXiv:2305.01937 (2023)
4. Ashok, D., Lipton, Z.C.: PromptNER: Prompting for named entity recognition. arXiv preprint arXiv:2305.15444 (2023)
5. Raman, K., Naim, I., Chen, J., Hashimoto, K., Yalasangi, K., Srinivasan, K.: Transforming sequence tagging into a seq2seq task. In: Proceedings of Conference on Empirical Methods in Natural Language Processing, Abu Dhabi, United Arab Emirates, pp. 11856–11874. Association for Computational Linguistics (2022)

6. Zhang, N., et al.: CBLUE: a Chinese biomedical language understanding evaluation benchmark. In: Proceedings of Annual Meeting of the Association for Compu-tational Linguistics (Volume 1: Long Papers), Dublin, Ireland, pp. 7888–7915. Associa-tion for Computational Linguistics (2022)

7. Zhu, W., Wang, X., Zheng, H., Chen, M., Tang, B.: PromptCBLUE: A chinese prompt tuning benchmark for the medical domain. arXiv preprint arXiv:2310.14151 (2023)

8. Zhu, W., et al.: Extracting decision trees from medical texts: an overview of the text2dt track in chip2022. In: Tang, B., et al. (ed.) Health Information Processing. Evaluation Track Papers. CHIP 2022 CCIS, vol. 1773, pp. 89–102. Springer, Singapore, pp. 89–102 (2022) https://doi.org/10.1007/978-981-99-4826-0_9

9. Zhu, W., Wang, X., Chen, M., Tang, B.: Overview of the promptCBLUE shared task in CHIP2023. arXiv preprint arXiv:2312.17522 (2023)

10. Brown, T., et al.: Language models are few-shot learners. In: Proceedings of Conference on Neural Information Processing Systems, Vancouver, Canada, pp. 1877–1901 (2020)

11. Lu, Y., Bartolo, M., Moore, A., Riedel, S., Stenetorp, P.: Fantastically ordered prompts and where to find them: overcoming few-shot prompt order sensitivity. In: Proceedings of Annual Meeting of the Association for Computational Linguistics (Volume 1: Long Papers), Dublin, Ireland, pp. 8086–8098. Association for Computational Linguistics (2022)

12. Rubin, O., Herzig, J., Berant, J.: Learning to retrieve prompts for in-context learning. In: Proceedings of Conference of the North American Chapter of the Association for Computational Linguistics: Human Language Technologies, Seattle, United States, pp. 2655–2671. Association for Computational Linguistics (2022)

13. Su, H., et al.: Selective annotation makes language models better few-shot learners. In: The International Conference on Learning Representations, Kigali, Rwanda, Africa, pp. 1–24 (2023)

14. Zhao, Z., Wallace, E., Feng, S., Klein, D., Singh, S.: Calibrate before use: Improving few-shot performance of language models. In: International Conference on Machine Learning, Vienna, Austria, pp. 12697–12706. Proceedings of Machine Learning Research (2021)

15. Wei, J., et al.: Emergent abilities of large language models. arXiv preprint arXiv:2206.07682 (2022)

16. Dong, Q., et al.: A survey for in-context learning. arXiv preprint arXiv:2301.00234 (2022)

17. Li, X., Qiu, X.: Finding support examples for in-context learning. arXiv preprint arXiv:2302.13539 (2023)

18. Liu, J., Shen, D., Zhang, Y., Dolan, B., Carin, L., Chen, W.: What makes good in-context examples for GPT-3?. In: Proceedings of Deep Learning Inside Out: The Workshop on Knowledge Extraction and Integration for Deep Learning Architectures, Dublin, Ireland and Online, pp. 100–114. Association for Computational Linguistics (2022)

19. Li, X., et al.: Unified demonstration retriever for in-context learning. arXiv preprint arXiv:2305.04320 (2023)

20. Min, S., et al.: Rethinking the role of demonstrations: what makes in-context learning work? In: Proceedings of Conference on Empirical Methods in Natural Language Processing, Abu Dhabi, United Arab Emirates, pp. 11048–11064. Association for Computational Linguistics (2022)

21. Olsson, C., et al.: In-context learning and induction heads. arXiv preprint arXiv:2209.11895 (2022)

22. Garg, S., Tsipras, D., Liang, P.S., Valiant, G.: What can transformers learn in-context? A case study of simple function classes. In: Proceedings of Conference on Neural Information Processing Systems, New Orleans, USA, pp. 30583–30598 (2022)

23. Fu, D., Chen, T., Jia, R., Sharan, V.: Transformers learn higher-order optimization methods for in-context learning: A study with linear models. arXiv preprint arXiv:2310.17086 (2023)
24. Reimers, N., Gurevych, I.: Sentence-BERT: Sentence embeddings using siamese BERT-networks. In: Proceedings of Conference on Empirical Methods in Natural Language Processing and the 9th International Joint Conference on Natural Language Processing, Hong Kong, China, pp. 3982–3992. Association for Computational Linguistics (2019)

Chinese Medical Text Few-shot Named Entity Recognition

CMF-NERD: Chinese Medical Few-Shot Named Entity Recognition Dataset with State-of-the-Art Evaluation

Chenghao Zhang, Yunlong Li , Kunli Zhang[✉], and Hongying Zan

School of Computer and Artificial Intelligence, Zhengzhou University,
Zhengzhou, Henan, China
{ieklzhang,iehyzan}@zzu.edu.cn

Abstract. Current works about medical few-shot named entity recognition (NER) predominantly focuses on English texts. There are also some supervised Chinese medical NER datasets available. The difficulty to share private data and varying specifications presented pose a challenge to this research. In this paper, We merged and cleaned multiple sources of Chinese medical NER dataset, then restructured these data into few-shot settings. CMF-NERD was constructed by weighted random sampling algorithm, containing 8,891 sentences and comprising 16 entity types. We adapted the most recent state-of-the-art few-shot learning methods and large language model for NER and conducted systematic experiments. The results indicate that the Chinese medical small-sample NER task is challenging and requires further research. Our further analysis provides promising directions for future studies.

Keywords: Chinese Medical Named Entity Recognition · Few-shot Learning · Dataset Construction

1 Introduction

Chinese medical named entity recognition is a foundational task for wise information technology of med, aims to extract disease, symptom, and treatment information within text. Deep neural networks and Transformer-based models have emerged as the mainstream methods for NER. However, when the number of trainable instances decreases to 50 or even fewer, there is a drastic performance decline in these models. This suggests that a limited number of instances is insufficient for the model to learn deep-level features.

In real-world scenarios. datasets with different languages, domains, and annotation styles are challenging to share. A well-trained model on one dataset may not yield satisfactory results when applied to another dataset. More research focuses on achieving high accuracy with minimal labeled data and ensuring the model possesses strong generalization capabilities.

Few-Shot Learning (FSL) [1], introduced in recent years, aims to address issues related to data scarcity and domain transfer. In 2021, Tsinghua University collaborated with Alibaba to complete the first few-shot entity recognition

H. Xu et al. (Eds.): CHIP 2023, CCIS 2080, pp. 87–97, 2024.
https://doi.org/10.1007/978-981-97-1717-0_7

dataset, Few-NERD [2]. The authors provided four types of N-way-K-shot tasks, where N represents the number of entity types in an episode, and K represents the number of instances each type. This open benchmark significantly propelled the research development in few-shot NER, giving rise to numerous methods represented by transfer learning, meta-learning, and data-driven approaches. Taking the example of 5-way-1-shot, over the past two years, the F1 evaluation metric for state-of-the-art models increased from 51.88 to 76.86 [3].

The quantity of resources such as electronic health records and medical literature continues to increase; however, due to the high privacy concerns surrounding medical data, it often cannot be used for public research. Constructing new high-quality datasets requires extensive professional annotation. Therefore, in the Chinese medical domain, there are only a few supervised datasets for public, which vary in granularity and consist of entity types ranging from 9 to 19. Treatment entities in one dataset might be categorized as drug, surgery, and other treatment in another dataset. Additionally, medical records often revolve around diseases, exhibiting a significant long-tail problem where the number of "disease" entities greatly surpasses the count of "surgical treatment" entities, sometimes differing by as much as tenfold [4]. These problems have hindered the progress of research in Chinese medical few-shot NER.

Therefore, we conducted systematic analysis and resampled multiple medical NER datasets, combining the characteristics of various entity systems. Then presented CMF-NERD, a Chinese medical text Few-shot entity recognition dataset, which originates from pediatric, obstetrics, cardiology, and oncology departments. We propose a weighted random sampling algorithm to balance the distribution of each entity type, resulting in the creation of two settings: 5-way-1-shot and 5-way-5-shot. In summary, the contributions of this paper are summarized as follows:

(1) We present a few-shot Chinese medical NER dataset, formulating Chinese medical NER as FSL task.
(2) We conducted experiments on state-of-the-art FSL models and established the benchmark for this dataset. This not only highlights the challenges within this domain but also indicates potential research directions.

2   Related Works

2.1   Few-Shot NER Datasets

Named entity recognition, as a common task in information extraction, has undergone over 20 years of development and now boasts a considerable number of supervised datasets encompassing various domains in both English and Chinese.The CoNLL03 dataset [5] is widely used for general Named Entity Recognition tasks in English; it includes four coarse-grained entity types. The ACE05 [6] and OntoNotes 5.0 [7] datasets contain Chinese texts primarily sourced from online resources such as news reports and conversations.

With the advancements in deep learning methods, supervised Named Entity Recognition has demonstrated desirable performance. More researchers are now directed towards challenging tasks like few-shot learning. Some works involve reorganizing supervised datasets into few-shot settings.However, these datasets often have few entity types, making it difficult to establish a unified evaluation standard. Few-NERD [2] is the first few-shot NER dataset with a large amount of manual annotation. Apart from this, there are few public benchmarks available.

2.2   Medical NER Datasets

In the medical domain, data requires higher expertise from annotators and often contains sensitive information, which limits open-source research within the academic community. PubMed is a large open-access medical database comprising over 32 million biomedical articles and abstracts, serving as a crucial source of English-language primary text in the field. Li et al. [8] annotated disease and drug entities from 1,500 abstracts in PubMed (BC5CDR dataset). The DDI [9] dataset is smaller, comprising only 792 instances sourced from a drug database. The ChemProt [10] dataset documents interactions between drugs and proteins, while BioRED [11] encompasses gene, disease, and drug entities simultaneously. ADE [12] is a benchmark corpus to extract drug-related adverse effects from medical case reports. Research on medical few-shot NER builds upon previous works. For instance, Li et al. [13] reformatted data from BC5CDR and NCBI into 1-shot and 5-shot formats, achieving peak performances of 91.28 and 90.79, respectively, on large language model(LLM). These datasets involve only a small number of medical entities found in real-life scenarios, thus achieving notably good performance.

Research on Chinese medical NER originated from electronic medical records (EMRs) and has been evolving towards finer-grained entity types. Yang et al. [14] identified diseases, disease diagnoses, symptoms, examinations, and treatments as primary entity types in clinical texts. They annotated named entities and relationships in 992 real medical records. Ye et al. [15], considering the specific format of electronic medical records for diabetes, incorporated temporal modifiers for diseases and symptoms. They constructed a corpus of entity relationships within electronic medical records for diabetes.Chang et al. [16], developed a corpus of entity relationships within electronic medical records for stroke and cardiovascular conditions. Wang et al. [17] introduced a label-aware dual-transfer learning framework for experiments in cross-domain few-shot NER. They utilized 1,600 electronic medical records from cardiology, respiratory, neurology, and gastroenterology as the target domains.

The China Conference on Knowledge Graph and Semantic Computing (CCKS) and the China Health Information Processing Conference (CHIP), organized by the Chinese Information Processing Society of China(CIPS), have published a series of information extraction tasks. Of which the CBLUE [18] benchmark introduced the CMeEE NER task, categorizing entities into 9 types: diseases, clinical manifestations, drugs, medical equipment, medical procedures, body, medical examinations, microorganisms, and department. Subsequently, the Trigger Entity Recognition dataset released during CHIP 2022 aimed to identify 12 types of molecular entities related to "gene-disease" associations along with their trigger entities. The CMedCasual dataset emphasizes capturing the premises of causality as entities, specifically designed for extracting condition-cause-effect relationships. For private datasets, there are mainly small to medium-sized datasets specific to particular diseases and departments, such as pediatrics [19], obstetrics [20], and Symptom Knowledge Base [21].

In conclusion, current research on medical few-shot NER primarily focuses on English datasets, although there are also some supervised Chinese medical NER datasets available.

3   CMF-NERD Dataset

3.1   Data Source

We focused on four Chinese medical NER datasets tailored for various diseases to analyze the characteristics of Chinese medical texts. These datasets, curated for different ailments, exhibit variations in their overall structures. Specifically, they encompass public datasets like CMeEE [18] and proprietary ones such as CPeKG [4], CIKG, and CvdKG.

CMeEE. This dataset was constructed from 504 pediatric medical textbooks and electronic health records, was introduced in the CHIP 2020 evaluation task. It categorizes named entities in medical texts into nine major classes: diseases (dis), clinical manifestations (sym), drugs (dru), medical equipment (equ), medical procedures (pro), anatomy (bod), medical examination items (ite), microorganisms (mic), and departments (dep).

CPeKG. Under medical supervision, medical knowledge, consisting of 26 entity types totaling 62,287 entities, was extracted using automated and semi-automated techniques from professional textbooks, national policies, diagnosis and treatment standards, clinical pathways, clinical practices and guidelines, as well as publicly available online resources. These entities primarily encompass diseases, symptoms, drugs, EEG (electroencephalogram) manifestations, and medical examinations.

CIKG. The authors annotated over 3.56 million words from electronic medical records and medical textbooks related to liver cancer, lung cancer, and breast cancer. Additionally, through web scraping techniques, they supplemented this data by collecting medical knowledge from various sources such as medical encyclopedias, disease encyclopedias, and the Chinese Disease Knowledge Library. This expanded dataset comprises 64,735 entities across 12 entity types, including diseases, symptoms, anatomical locations, examinations, treatments, sociology, epidemiology, and more.

CvdKG. The authors automatically extracted and validated knowledge from cardiovascular disease medical textbooks, clinical guidelines, and other texts.

They identified 15 core entity types centered around diseases and surgeries, comprising 217 core cardiovascular diseases, 8,845 related diseases, and 433 surgeries. This dataset can support intelligent cardiovascular disease querying and assistive diagnostics.

The aforementioned medical text datasets are mostly constructed from medical textbooks, which often result in longer sentences and fewer entities in some cases. This chapter begins by filtering sentences and entities within the datasets. Figure 1 illustrates the entity counts for each dataset after preprocessing.

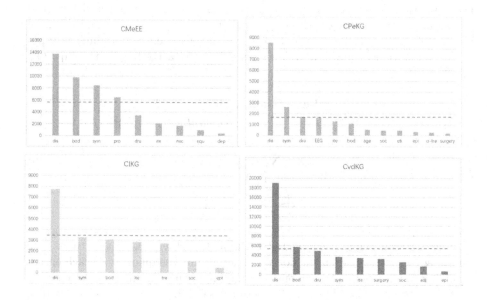

Fig. 1. Detailed statistics of medical NER datasets.

The dashed lines in the figure represent the average entity counts for each dataset. According to the information presented in Fig. 1, all four datasets exhibit a long-tail distribution, signifying data imbalance. Some entity types have significantly fewer instances compared to others, typically exceeding a tenfold difference, indicating an imbalance issue in the dataset. In such situations, the model will heavily favor types with a larger number of instances. This can lead to underfitting issues for the few-shot types, resulting in poor generalization and low robustness of the model.

3.2   Resampling and Analysis

To address the issue of imbalanced data, it's necessary to resample the data into few-shot settings. Unlike typical classification tasks, entities in medical texts are relatively dense, with each NER sentence containing multiple types of entities, making it hard to satisfy the N-way-K-shot settings. In previous work, entities outside of N types were labeled as 'O'. We believe this approach introduces more noise into the data. Therefore, we've adopted a more lenient sampling algorithm to balance data distribution as much as possible in few-shot settings. Specifically, we proposed a weighted random sampling algorithm, assigning a weight to each type. Subsequently, data was randomly sampled based on these weights, allowing a higher probability of sampling more important instances.

Given N medical entity types $L = l_1, l_2, \ldots, l_n$, we first calculate the number of entities for each type $Count_{l_i}$ in the Support Set or Query Set, each type needs at least K entities. For type l_i, the sampling weight w_{l_i} is determined by the number of missing entities z_{l_i} for that category in the set and the total number of entities Z. The sampling weight w for a sentence containing m types is the summation of multiple weights, as calculated according to the Eqs. (1), (2), and (3).

$$z_{l_i} = \begin{cases} K - Count_{l_i}, & Count_{l_i} < K \\ 0, & Count_{l_i} \geq K \end{cases} \tag{1}$$

$$Z = \sum_{i=1}^{N} z_{l_i}, w_i = \frac{z_{l_i}}{Z} \tag{2}$$

$$w = \sum_{i=1}^{m} w_{l_i}, m \leq K, l_i \in L \tag{3}$$

Repeated sampling is conducted to fulfill the N-way K-shot settings. The sampling method being lenient doesn't strictly limit the quantity of each entity. Sampling weights help avoid erroneous sampling, hence eliminating the need for post-sampling dataset filtering. The detailed sampling process is illustrated in Algorithm 1, comprising steps 1 to 7: Initialization stage, where for the sentence set X in the original dataset, its label set is denoted as Y. First, initialize the support set S and the query set Q as $\varnothing$ and compute the entity count for each type in the set. Then calculate the sampling weight w_{l_i} for each type and the weight of sentences in X. Steps 8 to 12: Sampling stage involves repeated sampling until the set S or Q meets the basic requirements of N-way-K-shot. Randomly select sentences based on weight w to add to the set, simultaneously updating the statistics and weights of each entity.

Based on the calculated weights during sampling, sentences containing relatively more types are prioritized for extraction. These sentences' context implies potential associative information among various similar entities. The N-way-K-shot settings can be achieved by sampling a small number of sentences, enhancing sampling efficiency. This method doesn't strictly limit the entity count to K, preserving the distribution characteristics of entities in the original data. Take train set for example, Fig. 2 illustrates the distribution of entities before and after sampling.

The integrated dataset comprises a total of 16 labels: item, sociology, disease, etiology, body, age, adjuvant therapy, electroencephalogram, equipment, drug,

---

Algorithm 1. Few-Shot NER Weighted Random Sampling algorithm

Input: Sentences X, Label Set Y, Parameters N, K
Output: Support Set S, Query Set Q
   //Initialize S, Q and the sampling weight w_j for each sentence.
1: $S \leftarrow \varnothing$, $S \leftarrow \varnothing$
2: **for** $i = 1$ in N **do**
3:   | $Count_{l_i} = 0$
4: **end for**
5: **for** $i = 1$ in N **do**
6:   | $w_i = \frac{z_{l_i}}{Z}$
7: **end for**
8: **for** $j = 1$ in $len(X)$ **do**
9:   | $w_j = \sum_{i=1}^{m} w_{l_i}$
10: **end for**

11: **repeat**
12:   | Randomly sample $(x, y, w) \in X$ that y includes l_i
13:   | Add (x, y, w) to S or Q
14:   | Update all $Count_{l_i}$, w_{l_i}, w_j //Update the sampled quantities and weights.
15:   | Update Dataset X
16: **until** $Count_{l_i} \geq K$

---

procedure, treatment, microorganism, department, epidemiology, and symptom. Common medical entities are used for training, while entities specific to scenarios like electroencephalogram, sociology, microorganism, are used to test the model's generalization ability. We've considered two few-shot experimental settings: 5-way-1-shot and 5-way-5-shot. Table 1 shows the results after sampling.

Table 1. Detailed statistics of CMF-NERD dataset.

Setting		Samples	sentences	types
5w1s	train	400	2960	'ite', 'soc', 'tre', 'bod', 'sym', 'dis', 'dep', 'dru'
	dev	100	964	'eti', 'EEG', 'age', 'adj', 'equ', 'mic', 'epi', 'dep'
	test	100	946	'eti', 'EEG', 'age', 'adj', 'equ', 'mic', 'epi', 'dep'
5w5s	train	400	14224	'ite', 'soc', 'tre', 'bod', 'sym', 'dis', 'dep', 'dru'
	dev	100	4707	'eti', 'EEG', 'age', 'adj', 'equ', 'mic', 'epi', 'dep'
	test	100	4707	'eti', 'EEG', 'age', 'adj', 'equ', 'mic', 'epi', 'dep'

4 Experiments

4.1 Task Formulation

NER is commonly modeled as a sequence labeling task. For each character $t_i \in S$ in an input sentence $S = t_1, t_2, \ldots, t_n$, assuming both the support set and query set contain a label set L_n of length N. Given an input sentence S and sets L_n containing K instances for each type, the objective is to find the optimal annotation sequence $Y = y_1, y_2, \ldots, y_n$ for S.

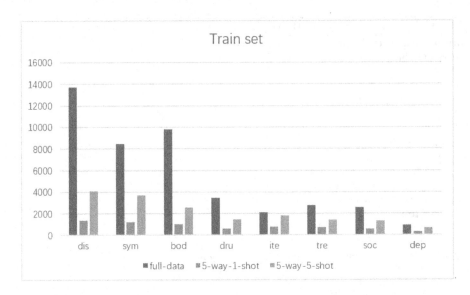

Fig. 2. Comparison of entity distribution in train set before and after sampling.

4.2   Baselines

We conducted experiments with several representative models on the CMF-NERD dataset, including methods based on meta-learning and prompt learning. For the Small Language Model(SLM), we utilized BERT-Base-Chinese as the pre-trained model. Here are the specifics:

ProtoBERT [22]. Prototypical network model utilizing BERT as encoder. As one of the representative meta-learning methods, its main idea is, representing data as a set of prototypes, where each prototype represents a centroid of a class or data distribution. During the meta-test phase, similarity between query instances (using Euclidean distance, cosine similarity, etc.) and prototypes is computed for classification.

NNShot [23]. This model considers NER as a sequence labeling task. It designs different neural network structures for the meta-learner and the base learner of the target task, using gradient descent algorithms for joint training.

DecomposedNER [3]. This model breaks down NER into two subtasks: span prediction and entity classification. It uses the MAML (Model-Agnostic Meta-Learning) algorithm to train a span predictor, aiming to find better initial model parameters.

WinGPT-7B-Base [24]. A GPT-based LLM in the medical domain which has been open-sourced to the community. This model is fine-tuned based on the Qwen-7B model, using a training corpus comprising a professional medical knowledge base and open-source data, totaling 500,000 instructions and 20 GB of

data. It outperforms various other 7B models on the Chinese benchmark evaluation C-EVAL. Considering the impact of prompt templates on results, we tested
the zero-shot performance of this model using 23 different NER instructions.

4.3   Results and Analysis

We evaluate these models by Precision (P), Recall (R), and F1 score. Precision
represents the proportion of entities predicted as medical entities that are truly
medical entities. Recall represents the proportion of all true medical entities
that are predicted as medical entities by the model. F1 score is the weighted
harmonic mean of Precision and Recall, providing a comprehensive evaluation
of the performance of few-shot NER models.

In Table 2, We reported the overall results. Based on the preliminary experiments, it appears that the CMF-NERD dataset presents certain challenges.
Early small-sample learning methods (ProtoBERT and NNShot) exhibited poor
performance. Even the state-of-the-art model (DecomposedNER) struggled on
this task, showing performance of 0.316 and 0.330 in the two settings. with the
boundary recognition notably lower than the classification performance. The
lower boundary recognition compared to classification performance is mainly
because most of entities in the test set being within long spans, making their
boundaries hard to determine. Even if the model has effectively learned the characteristics of the training set's types, it doesn't guarantee satisfactory results on
the test set. Additionally, WinGPT's performance in zero-shot setting surpasses
methods like NNshot, indicating that LLM holds significant potential in few-
shot learning. Determining the boundaries of long entities like "Entirely irregular
slow spike-wave or focal epileptiform abnormalities, often located in the occip-
ital region, with possible enlarged cortical evoked potentials" is an important
research direction in future.

Table 2. Experimental results of different models on CMF-NERD dataset.

Models	5-w-1-s			5-w-5-s		
	P	R	F1	P	R	F1
ProtoBERT	0.061	0.203	0.098	0.084	0.193	0.123
NNShot	0.098	0.158	0.142	0.134	0.207	0.162
DecomposedNER(Span)	0.378	0.447	0.410	0.322	0.449	0.375
DecomposedNER(Type)	0.747	0.747	0.747	0.840	0.840	0.840
DecomposedNER(Overall)	**0.291**	**0.345**	**0.316**	**0.284**	**0.395**	**0.330**
WinGPT	0.213	0.179	0.195	0.221	0.176	0.197

We also noticed that meta-learning methods tend to have a higher recall than
precision, indicating that these models incorrectly identified more entities. On
the other hand, LLM exhibits higher precision than recall, potentially due to

its vast domain-specific knowledge, making it better at distinguishing genuine entities from false ones. That's a possible approach–using meta-learning methods to extract candidate entity sets and then having LLM rank these results, returning the highest-scored entities. This approach could potentially improve the precision of the meta-learning methods to a certain extent.

5 Conclusion

"Chinese medical few-shot learning" is an urgently needed research area. In this paper, we integrate Chinese medical NER data from pediatrics, obstetrics, cardiology, and oncology, establishing a benchmark for NER tasks in few-shot settings. To address the imbalance in the original dataset, we proposed a weighted random sampling algorithm where entities with fewer instances were assigned higher sampling weights. The CMF-NERD we proposed comprises 8891 sentences and 16 entity types, following both the 5-way-1-shot and 5-way-5-shot settings. The experiments conducted on representative meta-learning methods and LLM demonstrate the inherent difficulty in the Chinese medical few-shot NER task. When the number of instances drastically decrease, models struggle to correctly identify entity boundaries. In future work, We will consider enhancing the modeling of entity boundaries and injecting more domain-specific knowledge into LLM to improve the existing methods.

Acknowledgments. We appreciate the constructive feedback from the anonymous reviewers and the support provided for this research by the following projects: Zhengzhou City Collaborative Innovation Major Projects (20XTZX11020), and the Science and Technology Innovation 2030-"New Generation of Artificial Intelligence" Major Project under Grant No. 2021ZD0111000.

References

1. Lake, B.M., Salakhutdinov, R., Tenenbaum, J.B.: Human-level concept learning through probabilistic program induction. Science **350**(6266), 1332–1338 (2015)
2. Ding, N., Xu, G., Chen, Y., et al.: Few-NERD: a few-shot named entity recognition dataset. In: Proceedings of the 59th Annual Meeting of the Association for Computational Linguistics and the 11th International Joint Conference on Natural Language Processing (Volume 1: Long Papers), pp. 3198–3213 (2021)
3. Dong, G., Wang, Z., Zhao, J., et al.: A multi-task semantic decomposition framework with task-specific pre-training for few-shot NER. In: Proceedings of the 32nd ACM International Conference on Information and Knowledge Management, pp. 430–440 (2023)
4. Zhang, K., Gao, Q., Zhang, J., et al.: construction of Chinese pediatric epilepsy knowledge graph. In: 2023 IEEE 36th International Symposium on Computer-Based Medical Systems (CBMS), pp. 241–244. IEEE (2023)
5. Sang, E.F., De Meulder, F.: Introduction to the CoNLL-2003 shared task: language-independent named entity recognition (2003). arXiv preprint cs/0306050

6. Walker, C., Strassel, S., Medero, J., et al.: ACE 2005 multilingual training corpus, Linguistic Data Consortium (2006). Web download: https://catalog.ldc.upenn. edu/LDC2006T06

7. Weischedel, R., Palmer, M., Marcus, M., et al.: Ontonotes release 5.0 ldc2013t19. Linguistic Data Consortium, Philadelphia, PA, 23 (2013)

8. Li, J., Sun, Y., Johnson, R.J., et al.: BioCreative V CDR task corpus: a resource for chemical disease relation extraction. Database, 2016 (2016)

9. Segura-Bedmar, I., Martínez Fernández, P., Herrero, Z.M.: Semeval-2013 task 9: extraction of drug-drug interactions from biomedical texts (ddiextraction 2013). Association for Computational Linguistics (2013)

10. Taboureau, O., Nielsen, S.K., Audouze, K., et al.: ChemProt: a disease chemical biology database. Nucleic Acids Res. **39**(suppl_1), D367–D372 (2010)

11. Luo, L., Lai, P.T., Wei, C.H., et al.: BioRED: a rich biomedical relation extraction dataset. Brief. Bioinform. **23**(5), bbac282 (2022)

12. Gurulingappa, H., Rajput, A.M., Roberts, A., et al.: Development of a benchmark corpus to support the automatic extraction of drug-related adverse effects from medical case reports. J. Biomed. Inform. **45**(5), 885–892 (2012)

13. Li, M., Zhang, R.: How far is Language Model from 100

14. Yang, J.F., et al.: Corpus construction for named entities and entity relations on Chinese electronic medical records. Ruan Jian Xue Bao J. Softw. **27**(11), 2725–2746 (2016)

15. Ye, Y., Hu, B., Zhang, K., et al.: Construction of corpus for entity and relation annotation of diabetes electronic medical records. In: Proceedings of the 20th Chinese National Conference on Computational Linguistics, pp. 622–632 (2021)

16. Chang, H., Zan, H., Ma, Y., et al.: Corpus construction for named-entity and entity relations for electronic medical records of stroke disease. In: Proceedings of the 20th Chinese National Conference on Computational Linguistics, pp. 633–642 (2021)

17. Wang, Z., Qu, Y., Chen, L., et al.: Label-aware double transfer learning for cross-specialty medical named entity recognition (2018). arXiv preprint arXiv:1804.09021

18. Zhang, N., Chen, M., Bi, Z., et al.: CBLUE: a Chinese biomedical language understanding evaluation benchmark (2021). arXiv preprint arXiv:2106.08087

19. Zan, H.Y., Liu, T., Niu, C.Y., Zhao, Y., Zhang, Y., Sui, Z.: Construction and application of named entity and entity relations corpus for pediatric diseases. J. Chin. Inf. Process. **34**(5), 19–26 (2020)

20. Zhang, K., Hu, C., Song, Y., et al.: Construction of Chinese obstetrics knowledge graph based on the multiple sources data. In: Dong, M., Gu, Y., Hong, J.F. (eds.) Chinese Lexical Semantics. CLSW 2021. LNCS, vol. 13250, pp. 399–410. Springer, Cham (2022). https://doi.org/10.1007/978-3-031-06547-7_31

21. Zan, H., Han, Y., Fan, Y., et al.: Construction and analysis of symptom knowledge base in Chinese. J. Chin. Inf. Process. **34**(4), 30–37 (2020)

22. Snell, J., Swersky, K., Zemel, R.: Prototypical networks for few-shot learning. Adv. Neural Inf. Process. Syst. **30** (2017)

23. Yang, Y., Katiyar, A.: Simple and effective few-shot named entity recognition with structured nearest neighbor learning. In: Proceedings of the 2020 Conference on Empirical Methods in Natural Language Processing (EMNLP), pp. 6365–6375, Online. Association for Computational Linguistics

24. https://github.com/winninghealth/WiNGPT2

Chinese Biomedical NER Based on Self-attention and Word-Relation Decoding Strategy

Wenxuan Mu, Di Zhao$^{(\boxtimes)}$, and Jiana Meng

School of Computer Science and Engineering, Dalian Minzu University,
Dalian 116000, Liaoning, China
{zhaodi,mengjn}@dlnu.edu.cn

Abstract. Biomedical named entity recognition plays a crucial role in advancing smart healthcare tasks. However, the scarcity of biomedical data and the extensive annotation required by professionals make achieving remarkable model performance challenging and expensive. Few-shot learning focuses on improving the model's performance and generalization under limited labeled data, providing effective solutions for biomedical information mining. Therefore, this paper proposes a Chinese biomedical named entity recognition method based on self-attention and word-relation decoding strategy. The aim is to effectively address the task of Chinese biomedical named entity recognition in few-shot scenarios. Our work is based on the 9th China Health Information Processing Conference task 2 and ranked third among all the teams. In the final results of the query set in the test dataset, the F1 score on testA dataset is 0.85, and on testB dataset, it is 0.87.

Keywords: Biomedical Named Entity Recognition · Few-Shot Learning · Self-Attention Mechanism · Word-Relation Decoding Strategy

1 Introduction

Due to the advancement of biomedical technology and the emergence of a large number of new literatures, a vast amount of medical information data has been generated. These datasets, with their challenging scale, make manual information extraction less practical. With continuous breakthroughs in Natural Language Processing (NLP), specific technologies and models have been developed, significantly enhancing the ability to automatically process biomedical text data. Among them, Biomedical Named Entity Recognition (BioNER) is a key technology, playing a crucial role as the foundation for various downstream tasks such as relationship extraction [1,2], knowledge graph construction [3], and question-answering systems [4,5]. BioNER aims to identify biomedical named entities in unstructured biomedical text and assign them to predefined entity types, such as genes, proteins, diseases, and chemical substances.

H. Xu et al. (Eds.): CHIP 2023, CCIS 2080, pp. 98–106, 2024.
https://doi.org/10.1007/978-981-97-1717-0_8

In recent years, deep learning methods [6] have garnered widespread attention across diverse research fields, owing to their capacity to automatically and effectively unveil hidden features. Notably, these methods have proven successful in the domain of BioNER. The typical architecture of a BioNER system comprises three key components: firstly, the encoder module, often leveraging BERT [7] and its various iterations to extract fundamental sentence representations; subsequently, the feature enhancement or fusion component, which integrates supplementary information or employs diverse machine learning methods to fortify feature representations. Examples include the incorporation of syntactic information [8,9], utilization of self-attention mechanisms [10], or the application of Conditional Random Fields (CRF) [6,9,11] to extract more insightful feature details. Lastly, the decoder or classifier is employed to recognize and categorize entities.

However, models based on deep learning architectures typically require a large amount of annotated data to exhibit good performance. Additionally, different task domains can significantly impact the model's performance, especially in the biomedical field. Moreover, data annotation in the biomedical domain remains a challenging task. Therefore, many BioNER studies are conducted directly in few-shot scenarios. These studies employ techniques such as data augmentation [12,13] and few-shot learning strategies to address the scarcity of annotated data.

In this work, we conducted an in-depth analysis of task 2 in CHIP-2023, which presented several challenges: (1) the entity types in the training set, validation set, and test set were mostly different, making it difficult for the model to learn knowledge about entity types in the test set. (2) The dataset was limited in quantity, requiring the model to extract valuable information as much as possible to enable rapid adaptation to new domains. (3) Entities in the data were generally lengthy, necessitating the model's ability to capture long-distance dependencies. (4) The dataset did not explicitly mention nested entity issues, and due to the presence of many long entities, it was crucial to avoid nested entity problems.

To address these challenges, we proposes a Chinese Biomedical NER Based on Self-Attention and Word-Relation Decoding Strategy. The model utilizes a two-dimensional grid structure [14] to represent word-relation, enhancing the representation space and allowing the model to capture knowledge as much as possible. This enables the model to efficiently handle new entity categories. Furthermore, the self-attention is introduced to effectively capture long-distance dependencies, capturing more useful features.

We reported experimental results under different data volumes, and the contributions are summarized as follows:

(1) We proposed a simple and effective model for BioNER.
(2) Our proposed method exhibited remarkable performance even in few-shot scenarios.
(3) Our model effectively captured feature information for new categories and demonstrated outstanding classification abilities.

2   Related Work

Traditional Named Entity Recognition (NER) tasks are typically treated as sequence labeling problems [15], where different labels are assigned to each token in a sentence based on different annotation strategies, such as the BIO labeling scheme, BIOES labeling scheme, etc. Given a text containing N tokens: $x_1, x_2, x_3, ..., x_N$, after passing it through the model, label information is obtained: $y_1, y_2, y_3, ..., y_N$, where x represents tokens, y represents labels, and N represents the sequence length. Mainstream methods often utilize machine learning and neural architectures, such as CNN [16,17], RNN, BiLSTM [18], CRF, Transformer [19,20], etc. Common frameworks usually employ $BERT + BiLSTM + CRF$ as the basic structure. However, these methods struggle to handle the issue of overlapping entities and have weak generalization capabilities.

Additionally, there are span-based approaches [10,21,22], which enumerates all possible spans and then determines whether these spans are entities and of what entity type. However, since this method enumerates all possibilities, when entities are generally long (e.g., in the biomedical domain), the number of enumerated spans will dramatically increase, leading to increased inference time.

In low-resource scenarios, few-shot learning is a promising strategy, including methods like data augmentation. However, due to restrictions on manipulating the dataset's content for this task, this methods cannot be effectively utilized. To address these challenges, this paper employs a two-dimensional grid structure for word relation decoding strategy, expanding the model's feature representation dimension while solving the problem of nested entities. This approach avoids enumeration problems and expands the representation information to capture features in low-resource scenarios as much as possible. Then, self-attention is used to capture more representative feature representations. Finally, a classifier is employed to recognize entities.

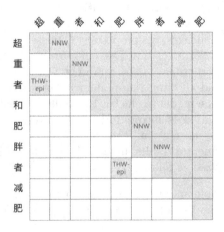

Fig. 1. Word-relation decoding strategy.

3   The Method

In this section, the decoding strategy of the model is presented first, followed by the overall framework of the model. Figure 1 shows a detailed presentation of the decoding strategy and Fig. 2 shows the overall framework of the model.

3.1   Overall Architecture

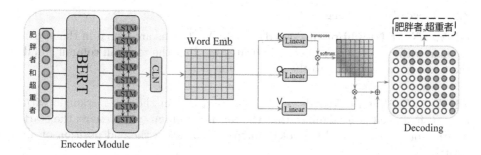

Fig. 2. The overall architecture of the model.

Encoder. As shown in the Fig. 2, first, the sentence $X = \{x_1, x_2, x_3, ..., x_n\}$ is input into the Bert encoder to get the contextual representation embedding $T = \{t_1, t_2, t_3, ..., t_n\}$. Then BiLSTM is utilized to extract the features $L = \{l_1, l_2, l_3, ..., l_N\}$. The formula is as follows:

$$t_1, t_2, ..., t_n = BERT(X) \tag{1}$$

$$l_1, l_2, ..., l_n = BiLSTM(T) \tag{2}$$

where $X \in \mathbb{R}^N$, $T \in \mathbb{R}^{N \times d}$, and $L \in \mathbb{R}^{N \times h}$. Here, N is the length of the sentence, d is the number of nodes in the hidden layer of the Bert encoder (usually 768 or 1024), and h is the number of nodes in the hidden layer of BiLSTM.

Self-attention Mechanism. After obtaining the context features through the above formulas, then using dimension expansion, the features $G \in \mathbb{R}^{N \times N \times h}$ in the form of a two-dimensional grid representation are obtained. Then the attention features $GA \in \mathbb{R}^{N \times N \times h}$ are obtained through the self-attention mechanism, and the $U \in \mathbb{R}^{N \times N \times 2h}$ is obtained by concatenating with the original features. Finally, through the classifiers and decoders, the entities are recognized. The formula is as follows:

$$G = Expand(T) \tag{3}$$

$$GA = Attention(G) \tag{4}$$

$$U = Concatenation([GA; G]) \tag{5}$$

The traditional use of the self-attention mechanism is to act on the features whose dimension is [b,len,emb], which has the advantages of fewer parameters, faster, more effective, and higher interpretable. And when acting on features whose dimensions are [b,len,len,emb], (1) it can better capture long-distance dependencies. (2) Contextual information can be captured more fully. (3) It can capture the features of all the tokens in the same sentence for each token.

3.2 Decoding Strategy

NNW (Next-Neighboring-Word). In NNW, tokens are stored in the upper triangle with $i < j$. Each cell (i, j) indicates whether the token in column j and the token in row i belong to the same entity.

THW-* (Tail-Head-Word-*). THW-* is stored in the lower triangle with $i >= j$. Each cell (i, j) signifies that the token in column j represents the start position of an entity, and the token in row i represents the end position of an entity.

As illustrated in Fig. 1, "超重者" and "肥胖者" are two entities. Taking "超重者" as an example, the NNW of "超" is "重", and the NNW of "重" is "者". The same applies to "肥胖者". Additionally, as "超重者" starts with "超" and ends with "者", in row 3 (where "者" is located), corresponding to column 1 (where "超" is located), the label is THW-epi at position $(3, 1)$, where "epi" represents the entity category. This decoding strategy allows us to obtain the final entities. The advantages of employing this decoding strategy are:

1. It effectively resolves entity nesting issues.
2. By expanding one dimension, the feature space transforms from n to n^2, providing more space to comprehensively capture features.

4 Experience

4.1 Dataset

The dataset is from the Natural Language Processing Laboratory, Zhengzhou University and integrates medical data from various sources, encompassing pediatric ailments, obstetrics and gynecology, cardiovascular conditions, and major diseases such as lung, liver, and breast cancers. Two settings in few-shot scenarios are given: 5-way-1-shot and 5-way-5-shot. Each set comprises 600 data pieces with five types in each. The data pieces have been sampled as per category distribution to minimize the amount of data since there is at least one sample from each category in the training set. The dataset is split into a training set, validation set, and test set in a 4:1:1 ratio, with each data stored in JSON format. The data comprises two subsets, support and query, featuring various medical sentences with labels of entities in the sequence annotation format. Table 1 provides specific quantitative and categorical data on the dataset.

Table 1. Dataset details

Setting	Dataset	Samples	Sentences	Entity Types
5	Train	400	2960	ite', 'soc','tre','bod','sym','dis','dep','dru'
w	Dev	100	964	eti','EEG','age','adj','equ','mic','epi','dep'
1	TestA	100	946	eti','EEG','age','adj','equ','mic','epi','dep'
s	TestB	100	942	eti','EEG','age','adj','equ','mic','epi','dep'
5	Train	400	14224	ite', 'soc','tre','bod','sym','dis','dep','dru'
w	Dev	100	4707	eti','EEG','age','adj','equ','mic','epi','dep'
5	TestA	100	4707	eti','EEG','age','adj','equ','mic','epi','dep'
s	TestB	100	4665	eti','EEG','age','adj','equ','mic','epi','dep'

4.2 Implementation Details

In this paper, we utilize `bert-base-chinese` as the encoder and access a hidden layer behind it as a 768-dimensional BiLSTM. The optimizer used is Adam, with Bert's learning rate set to 1×10^{-5} and the other learning rates set to 5×10^{-3}. The batch size is set to 12, the dropout to 0.5, and the epoch number to 40. We select and save the model parameters with the best F1 values on the validation set. The experiment was conducted using an NVIDIA GeForce RTX 3090 graphics card with 24 GB of memory.

4.3 Evaluation

According to the requirements of the competition, we have used the Macro-F1 value as the evaluation metric for this task. Its formula is as follows:

$$P_i = TP_i/(TP_i + FP_i) \tag{6}$$

$$R_i = TP_i/(TP_i + FN_i) \tag{7}$$

$$Macro - F1 = \frac{1}{N}\sum_{i=1}^{N}\frac{2 \cdot P_i \cdot R_i}{P_i + R_i} \tag{8}$$

Where P represents the accuracy rate, R represents the recall rate, and i in P_i and R_i represents the index of different entity types. The final score is calculated as the reconciled average of $Macro - F1$ for 5w1s and 5w5s.

4.4 Main Results

According to the data given in the task, the main results of the experiments in this paper are shown in Table 2. It can be seen that our method greatly outperforms traditional methods. And comparing the results of different pre-trained models, thanks to the adequate word representation of BERT-Large, the model is further improved.

Table 2. Online score results

Method	Score of testA(%)	Score of testB(%)
BERT	0.63	0.66
BERT+CRF	0.71	0.73
ours	0.85	0.87

In addition, we also conducted an ablation study, and the results of two experiments after using the overall architecture and removing the attention mechanism are shown in Table 3. We can see that after removing the attention mechanism, our model shows a decrease on both test sets, proving that the attention mechanism can effectively improve the performance of the model, which makes the model obtain an excellent result.

Table 3. Ablation experiments

Method	Score of testA(%)	Score of testB(%)
All	0.85	0.87
-Attention	0.81	0.84

5   Conclusion

In this paper, we proposed a Chinese biomedical NER model based on self-attention and word-relation decoding strategy, which utilises a feature representation of a 2D grid structure and the corresponding decoding strategy as well as the attention mechanism to extract and classify entities in Chinese biomedical texts in few-shot scenarios. The framework overcomes the problems of insufficient feature representation captured by the model in few-shot scenarios; the difficulty of capturing long-distance sentence features; and the problem of entity nesting. And the effectiveness of the model is experimentally verified while achieving remarkable performance.

References

1. Bach, N., Badaskar, S.: A review of relation extraction. Lit. Rev. Lang. Stat. **II**(2), 1–15 (2007)
2. Leng, J., Jiang, P.: A deep learning approach for relationship extraction from interaction context in social manufacturing paradigm. Knowl.-Based Syst. **100**, 188–199 (2016)
3. Li, L., et al.: Real-world data medical knowledge graph: construction and applications. Artif. Intell. Med. **103**, 101817 (2020)
4. Allam, A., Haggag, M.: The question answering systems: a survey. Int. J. Res. Rev. Inf. Sci. (IJRRIS) **2**(3) (2012)

5. Mishra, A., Jain, S.: A survey on question answering systems with classification. J. King Saud Univ. Comput. Inf. Sci. **28**(3), 345–361 (2016)
6. Dang, T., Le, H., Nguyen, T., Vu, S.: D3NER: biomedical named entity recognition using CRF-biLSTM improved with fine-tuned embeddings of various linguistic information. Bioinformatics **34**(20), 3539–3546 (2018)
7. Devlin, J., Chang, M., Lee, K., Toutanova, K.: BERT: pre-training of deep bidirectional transformers for language understanding. In: Burstein, J., Doran, C., Solorio, T. (eds.) Proceedings of the 2019 Conference of the North American Chapter of the Association for Computational Linguistics: Human Language Technologies, vol. 1, pp. 4171–4186. Association for Computational Linguistics (2019). https://doi.org/10.18653/v1/N19-1423
8. Tian, Y., Shen, W., Song, Y., Xia, F., He, M., Li, K.: Improving biomedical named entity recognition with syntactic information. BMC Bioinform. **21**(1), 1–17 (2020)
9. Li, D., Yan, L., Yang, J., Ma, Z.: Dependency syntax guided BERT-BiLSTM-GAM-CRF for Chinese NER. Expert Syst. Appl. **196**, 116682 (2022)
10. Yamada, I., Asai, A., Shindo, H., Takeda, H., Matsumoto, Y.: LUKE: deep contextualized entity representations with entity-aware self-attention. In: Webber, B., Cohn, T., He, Y., Liu, Y. (eds.) Proceedings of the 2020 Conference on Empirical Methods in Natural Language Processing (EMNLP), pp. 6442–6454. Association for Computational Linguistics (2020). https://doi.org/10.18653/v1/2020.emnlp-main.523
11. Lafferty, J., McCallum, A., Pereira, F.: Conditional random fields: probabilistic models for segmenting and labeling sequence data. In: Proceedings of the Eighteenth International Conference on Machine Learning, pp. 282–289. Morgan Kaufmann Publishers Inc (2001). Not Available
12. Liu, L., Ding, B., Bing, L., Joty, S., Si, L., Miao, C.: MulDA: a multilingual data augmentation framework for low-resource cross-lingual NER. In: Proceedings of the 59th Annual Meeting of the Association for Computational Linguistics and the 11th International Joint Conference on Natural Language Processing, vol. 1, pp. 5834–5846 (2021)
13. Ding, B., et al.: DAGA: data augmentation with a generation approach for low-resource tagging tasks. In: Webber, B., Cohn, T., He, Y., Liu, Y. (eds.) Proceedings of the 2020 Conference on Empirical Methods in Natural Language Processing (EMNLP), pp. 6045–6057. Association for Computational Linguistics (2020). https://doi.org/10.18653/v1/2020.emnlp-main.488
14. Li, J., et al.: Unified named entity recognition as word-word relation classification. In: Proceedings of the AAAI Conference on Artificial Intelligence, pp. 10965–10973 (2022)
15. Finkel, J., Grenager, T., Manning, C.: Incorporating Non-local Information into Information Extraction Systems by Gibbs Sampling. In: Proceedings of the 43rd Annual Meeting of the Association for Computational Linguistics, pp. 363–370 (2005)
16. Collobert, R., Weston, J., Bottou, L., Karlen, M., Kavukcuoglu, K., Kuksa, P.: Natural language processing (almost) from scratch. J. Mach. Learn. Res. **12**, 2493–2537 (2011)
17. Strubell, E., Verga, P., Belanger, D., McCallum, A.: Fast and accurate entity recognition with iterated dilated convolutions. In: Palmer, M., Hwa, R., Riedel, S. (eds.) Proceedings of the 2017 Conference on Empirical Methods in Natural Language Processing, pp. 2670–2680. Association for Computational Linguistics (2017). https://doi.org/10.18653/v1/D17-1283

18. Lample, G., Ballesteros, M., Subramanian, S., Kawakami, K., Dyer, C.: Neural architectures for named entity recognition. In: Knight, K., Nenkova, A., Rambow, O. (eds.) Proceedings of the 2016 Conference of the North American Chapter of the Association for Computational Linguistics: Human Language Technologies, pp. 260–270. Association for Computational Linguistics (2016). https://doi.org/10.18653/v1/N16-1030
19. Yan, H., Deng, B., Li, X., Qiu, X.: TENER: adapting transformer encoder for named entity recognition. ArXiv (2019)
20. Li, X., Yan, H., Qiu, X., Huang, X.: FLAT: Chinese NER using flat-lattice transformer. In: Jurafsky, D., Chai, J., Schluter, N., Tetreault, J. (eds.) Proceedings of the 58th Annual Meeting of the Association for Computational Linguistics, pp. 6836–6842. Association for Computational Linguistics (2020). https://doi.org/10.18653/v1/2020.acl-main.611
21. Xu, M., Jiang, H., Watcharawittayakul, S.: A local detection approach for named entity recognition and mention detection. In: Barzilay, R., Kan, M. (eds.) Proceedings of the 55th Annual Meeting of the Association for Computational Linguistics, vol. 1, pp. 1237–1247. Association for Computational Linguistics (2017). https://doi.org/10.18653/v1/P17-1114
22. Luan, Y., Wadden, D., He, L., Shah, A., Ostendorf, M., Hajishirzi, H.: A general framework for information extraction using dynamic span graphs. In: Burstein, J., Doran, C., Solorio, T. (eds.) Proceedings of the 2019 Conference of the North American Chapter of the Association for Computational Linguistics: Human Language Technologies, Volume 1 (Long and Short Papers), pp. 3036–3046. Association for Computational Linguistics (2019). https://doi.org/10.18653/v1/N19-1308

Drug Paper Document Recognition and Entity Relation Extraction

CHIP 2023 Task Overview: Complex Information and Relation Extraction of Drug-Related Materials

Qian Chen[✉], Jia Wang, Jia Xu, and Bingxiang Ji

Sinopharm Group Digital Technology (Shanghai) Co., Ltd., Shanghai, China
chenqian60@sinopharm.com

Abstract. Drug labels or package insert are legal documents that include significant information and are highly valuable. However, it contains both structured and unstructured information, which is challenging to extract. We construct a drug package insert information extraction dataset, which consists of 1,000 electronic files with a total of 17,000 structured fields and 24,580 entity relationships annotated. It is used in the CHIP2023 "Complex Information and Relation Extraction of Drug-related Materials" evaluation competition, in order to promote the development of printed material recognition and entity relationship extraction technology. Participants need to recognize structured fields from dataset and extract entity relationship from specified fields. Finally, we provide a concise overview and outline of their methods and discuss the potential value of the dataset in further study.

Keywords: Visual Document Understanding · Document Information Extraction · Optical Character Recognition · relation extraction

1 Introduction

An extensive collection of health-related data is becoming increasingly accessible to the scholarly community, corporate entities, and government departments. Specifically, healthcare practitioners can gather data from a variety of sources, including printed publications, literature databases, and online resources [1].

As such, practitioners engaged in the development of health information processing and applications sometimes may encounter the issue of an excessive number of resources from which to choose. Drug labels or package insert (PI), is an important source of health information for practitioners, yet it is sometimes overlooked. The PI is often an ideal resource for practitioners due to its accessibility, user-friendliness, thoroughness, and legal standing.

Nearly all pharmaceuticals introduced to the market are subject to specified regulations. The National Medical Products Administration (NMPA) implemented the latest requirements for PI on June 1, 2006 [2].

According to regulations, PI must have substantial evidence. NMPA reviews and approves data and their related evidence from the manufacturer before it can be added to the PI. A manufacturer can also take the initiative in changing PI to support a new indication or to raise a caution. The modified data must be inspected and approved by the NMPA as well [3]. The current PI format contains certain information about the drug, arranged in a specific format (Table 1) [4].

Table 1. Content of the Instructions for Chemical drugs

Specific information includes the following in the order listed:
- [Drug name]
- [Ingredients]
- [Description]
- [Indications]
- [Specification]
- [Usage and dosage]
- [Adverse reactions]
- [Contraindication]
- [Warnings and precautions]
- [Specific use for pregnant and nursing women]
- [Specific use for pediatrics]
- [Specific use for geriatrics]
- [Drug interactions]
- [Drug overdosage]
- [Clinical studies]
- [Pharmacology and toxicology]
- [Pharmacokinetics]
- [Storage]
- [Packaging]
- [Validity period]
- [Executive standard]
- [Approval No.]
- [Manufacturer]

However, it is important to note that despite the numerous regulations, the format of drug PI from various manufacturers are often not consistent, and changes with different printing layout, causing many useful information on PI to be unavailable. Some information hidden in PI also exist in an unstructured form, which cannot be used effectively. Mahatme [5] et al., have evaluated 270 package inserts and found that the information provided in most of them are not uniform. 5 They have pointed out that despite these regulatory and enforcing authorities, more than 10% of package inserts lacks information on pregnancy and lactation effects of drugs. Shivkar [6] noted, after studying 92 inserts, that information on interactions and overdose missing in most. Only five inserts have information on commonly encountered side effects.

2 Related Works

At present, researchers and corporate entities have proposed a number of methods to establish datasets of drug labels and PI, such as Zou [7] et al. proposed a method to build PI database in hospital, and Wan [8] proposed the creation of a commercial database containing details regarding twenty thousand medications. However, these databases still have insufficient coverage and lack extraction of structured fields. Therefore, this paper fully utilized the real-world data to construct a comprehensive dataset of PI and released the "Complex Information and Relation Extraction of Drug-related Materials" task on the CHIP2023 conference. Researchers can exploit the dataset to conduct research for entity relationship extraction, thus facilitating the advancement of drug-related printed material information extraction.

3 Dataset

3.1 Task Definition

This dataset is composed of real-world data, thus resulting in a wide variety of formats, layout, and printing quality. The dataset contains 1000 samples, each one an electronic file of a PI, and each sample may contain one or multiple pages.

The task involves recognizes structured fields from each sample and extracting the core entities from specified fields. The selection of structured fields is under NMPA's regulations (Table 2), while entity relationships extraction includes the following types. (Table 3).

Table 2. Structured Fields

1	Drug name
2	Trade name
3	Specification
4	Ingredients
5	Indications
6	Description
7	Usage and dosage
8	Adverse reactions
9	Contraindication
10	Warnings and precautions
11	Drug interactions
12	Specific use for pregnant and nursing women
13	Specific use for pediatrics
14	Specific use for geriatrics
15	Pharmacology and Toxicology
16	Pharmacokinetics
17	Storage

Table 3. Definition of Entity Relationship

relation_type	subtype	definition
drug_disease	indication	Refers to the application of drugs to certain diseases
drug_disease	contraindication	Refers to the inappropriate or prohibited use of drugs for certain diseases, which can cause serious adverse consequences
drug_disease	adverse_reaction	Refers to diseases unrelated to the purpose of treatment caused by the normal use of drugs for prevention, diagnosis, or treatment
drug_clinical_finding	indication	Refers to the application of drugs to certain symptoms or signs
drug_clinical_finding	contraindication	Refers to the inappropriate or prohibited use of drugs for certain symptoms or signs, which can cause serious adverse consequences
drug_clinical_finding	adverse_reaction	Refers to the occurrence of harmful reactions unrelated to the purpose of treatment caused by the normal use of drugs for prevention, diagnosis, or treatment
drug_drug	interaction	Refers to the compound effects that may occur after taking other drugs simultaneously, which can enhance the efficacy or reduce side effects, as well as weaken the efficacy or cause unexpected toxic side effects
drug_drug	additive_effect	Refers to the effect produced by combining with other drugs being equal to or close to the sum of the effects produced by separate applications
drug_drug	synergy	Refers to when used in combination with other drugs, the effect of mutual enhancement is achieved
drug_drug	antagonism	Refers to the weakening or disappearance of the effects produced by the combined use of other drugs,
drug_drug	incompatibility	Refers to the phenomenon where physical or chemical interactions directly occur when a drug is compatible in vitro, affecting its therapeutic effect or causing toxic reactions

3.2 Data Annotation

This task was headed by an experienced medical AI product expert, who provided four annotators with a two-hour instruction on the principles of annotation. All annotators work full-time at the authors' organization and have a background in the medical domain to conduct the annotation tasks. The task was based on the open source doccano labeling tool. We divided annotators into two groups, with 100 duplicate data between each group to calculate annotation agreement. We calculated micro f1 and macro f1 to measure the agreements, and the outcome was 0.854 and 0.877 respectively, which may be due to the use of paddle-uie for auto-labeling during the annotation process. Finally, a total of 24580 triplets were extracted from 1000 sample data, including 5679 indications, 1675 contraindications, 11974 adverse reactions, and 5252 drug interactions. The dataset was split into training, test A, and test B groups which have 400, 200, and 400 samples respectively.

3.3 Evaluation Metric

The task is evaluated using both average-cer and macro-f1. Considering the complexity of the task, the weighted score of the two indicators is used as the final metric. Score is calculated as follows:

$$Score = 0.3 \times (1 - \text{Average-CER}) + 0.7 \times \text{Macro-F1}$$

(1) **Average-CER:** Average CER of all structured fields. Each field's CER means the edit-distance between the predicted value and correct value of the specified field, divided by the total word number of the correct value. When both predicted value and correct value are "none", this value will not be included in the calculation.

(2) **Macro-F1:** Assuming that there are n categories, C_1, C_i, C_n, the calculation formula is as follows: Let the number of samples correctly predicted as category C_i be $T_{p(i)}$, the number of samples predicted as C_i is T_i, and the real The number of samples of C_i is P_i.

$$Precision_i = \frac{T_{p(i)}}{T_i}$$

$$Recall_i = \frac{T_{p(i)}}{P_i}$$

$$Macro - F1 = \frac{1}{n}\sum_{i=1}^{n}\frac{2 \times Precision_i \times Recall_i}{Precision_i + Recall_i}$$

4 Submission Result

4.1 Overall Statistics

The shared task is divided into two phases: the preliminary round (Round A) and the final round (Round B). The statistical result was shown in Table 4.

Table 4. Overall statistical result of the two rounds

Phase	Teams	Max	Min	Avg	Med	Std
Round A	8	0.2913	0.0000	0.0841	0.0652	0.0893
Round B	6	0.28	0	0.0767	0.0450	0.0970

4.2 Top Model

Table 5 shows the score of the top one in this evaluation. And we will give a brief introduction to their methods.

Table 5. Top score

Ranking	Organization	Max	Min	Avg	Med	Std
1st	8	0.2913	0.0000	0.0841	0.0652	0.0893

The first team preprocess the data, then use the DONUT model for structured extraction, which is better than using the DONUT model directly. After that, the team use a pre-trained entity extraction model UIE to extract medical knowledge tuples, and built an entity type dictionary based on the training data to post process the prediction results.

5   Conclusion

This paper summarizes the construction process of the PI dataset and the models and performance of participating teams. The dataset contains real-world image data, structured fields and entity relationships. The top team used rules, preprocessing and other methods to improve the performance. In general, the dataset is quite complex, presenting a significant challenge, and it is valuable for further study in the development and improvement of medical information extraction technologies.

References

1. JP Nathan, E Vider. The Package Insert[J]. U.S. Pharmacist, 2015, 40(5):8–15
2. 国家食品药品监督管理局.药品说明书和标签管理规定[J].中华人民共和国国务院公报, 2007, 8(09):4–5
3. 国家食品药品监督管理局.关于加强《药品说明书和标签管理规定》实施工作的通知:国食药监办[2007]311号.2007
4. 国家食品药品监督管理局.关于印发化学药品和生物制品说明书规范细则的通知:国食药监注[2006]202号.2006
5. Mahatme, M., Dakhale, G., Hiware, S., Wankhede, S., Salve, A., Mahatme, S.: Comparison of Indian package inserts in public and private sector: an urgent need for self-regulation. Int. J. Basic Clin. Pharmacol. **2**(2), 165 (2013)

6. Shivkar, Y.M.: Clinical information in drug package inserts in India. J. Postgrad. Med. **55**(2), 104 (2009)

7. 邹晓华,冯友根.在医院计算机网络上建立药品说明书数据库及其应用[J].中国现代应用药学, 2005, 22(4):3

8. 万众.人卫临床助手、人卫用药助手专业版上线科学诊疗和合理用药的好帮手[J].中国卫生信息管理杂志, 2019, 16(1):120.s

Rule-Enhanced Pharmaceutical Instructions Information Extraction Based on Deep Learning

Xiaodan Lv[1] , Ben Teng[2] , Haitao Zhang[3] , and Bo An[4(✉)]

[1] Yuanbao Kechuang Technology Co., Ltd, Beijing, China
[2] Beijing Shoebill Technology Co., Ltd., Beijing, China
[3] Department of Critical Care Medicine, Shanghai East Hospital,
Tongji University School of Medicine, Shanghai, China
[4] The Institute of Ethnology and Anthropology,
Chinese Academy of Social Sciences, Beijing, China
anbo724@163.com

Abstract. Pharmaceutical instructions information extraction is to transform the core content of drug manuals into formatted data, including entity recognition and relationship extraction, which is an essential value for rational drug use and drug management. The task is challenging due to the various formats of drug manuals and the noise of watermarks and stamps on the original images. For this reason, this paper proposes the Rule-enhanced Drug Description Information Extraction based on deep learning method, which is a pipeline-based method that includes three steps of data preprocessing, text recognition and sorting, and information extraction. The results of the CHIP2023-Recognition and Entity Relationship Extraction of Pharmaceutical Instruction task show that the method proposed in this paper is able to extract the information embedded in pharmaceutical instructions more effectively, and achieves first place in this evaluation. Significantly, it achieves the first place in the evaluation and is significantly better than the second place. However, there are obvious things that could be improved in this method, as the pipeline approach contains many different modules and processing steps, which makes optimization very difficult. In the future, we try end-to-end extraction of pharmaceutical instruction information on the basis of multimodal large models.

Keywords: Pharmaceutical Instructions · Information Extraction · Pipelines

1 Introduction

Pharmaceutical instructions act as statutory documents that encapsulate crucial information about medications, thereby serving as a guideline for accurately selecting pharmaceuticals, signifying their substantial value [10]. The process of extracting relationships between drugs and other entities from unstructured textual content, powering the crafting of comprehensive medical knowledge maps, is indispensable. This approach amplifies the efficacy of downstream tasks, inclusive of prescription audits, diagnostic assistance, and the promotion of patient health education.

By structuring the pharmaceutical instructions, data formats such as the knowledge graph of pharmaceutical instructions can support rational drug use judgment and promote drug safety. Through intelligent dialogue or Q&A methods [7], it further educates the public about the value and role of medicines.

However, the update frequency of pharmaceutical instructions often exceeds that of typical corpus sources, such as clinical treatment guidelines and medical textbooks, and they are more challenging to extract. Although the content included in pharmaceutical instructions from different manufacturers is similar, there are many differences in their format, containing both structured and unstructured information. Figure 1 presents an example of a pharmaceutical instruction.

Additionally, due to the diverse formats of pharmaceutical instruction manuals, including images, PDF files, and other data formats, structuring these instruction manuals mainly involves manual disassembly. This is not only time-consuming and labor-intensive but also requires the staff to have solid medical knowledge [8].

In response to this issue, this paper presents a pipeline-based method for extracting knowledge from pharmaceutical instruction manuals that can handle real data such as images and PDFs. Specifically, this method includes preprocessing, a text block analysis module, and knowledge extraction based on joint learning. The experimental results show that the method of pharmaceutical instruction entity recognition and relationship extraction proposed in this paper can effectively carry out the extraction of pharmaceutical instruction manuals. It won first place in the CHIP2023-Recognition and Entity Relationship Extraction of Pharmaceutical Instruction task[1], with a macro-F1 value of 0.21. The main reason for the suboptimal performance is due to the complexity of the input data quality.

The main contribution of this paper is that it provides a strong baseline for knowledge extraction in real-life scenarios of pharmaceutical instruction manuals. It helps to drive the task of knowledge extraction from pharmaceutical instruction manuals, offering a foundation for future research and work. This baseline allows subsequent researchers to build upon it for more in-depth and extensive exploration.

2   Method

The structuring of a pharmaceutical instruction manual includes several subtasks. First, it involves converting data from images and PDFs into pure text, followed by corresponding information extraction. This paper proposes a rule-enhanced pipeline extraction method, which mainly includes a preprocessing

---

[1] http://www.cips-chip.org.cn/.

module, a text recognition module, and information extraction module. The overall framework of this method is shown in Fig. 2, and this section will detail the content of each module.

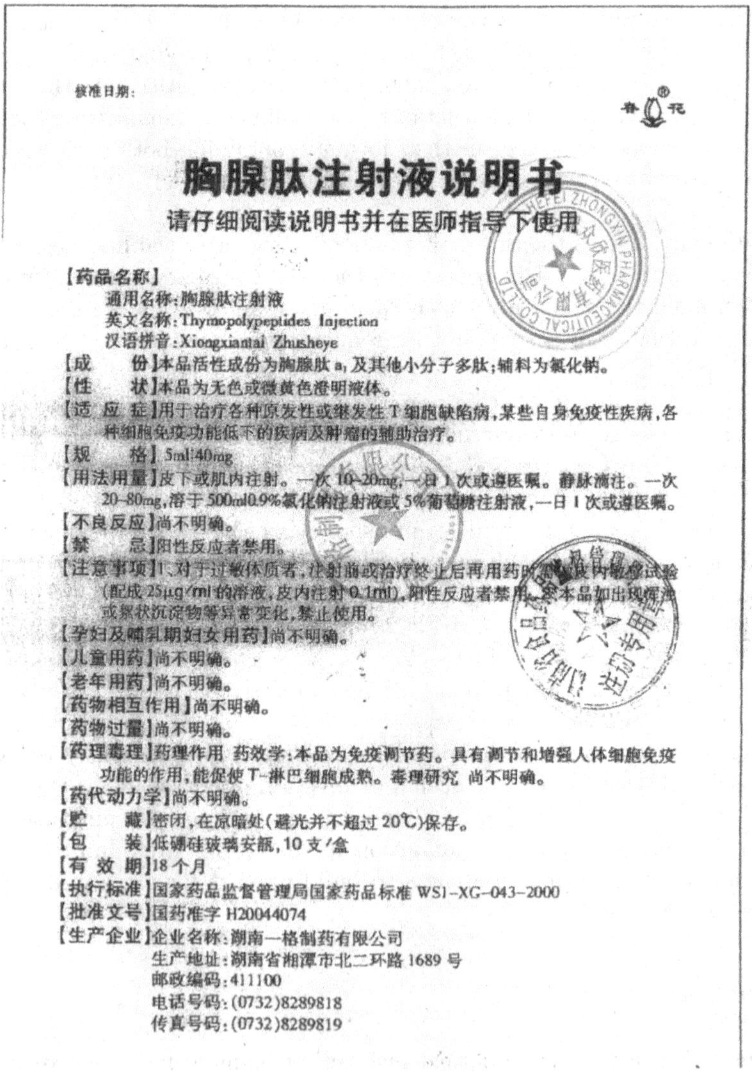

核准日期:

胸腺肽注射液说明书

请仔细阅读说明书并在医师指导下使用

【药品名称】
通用名称:胸腺肽注射液
英文名称:Thymopolypeptides Injection
汉语拼音:Xiongxiantai Zhusheye
【成　　份】本品活性成份为胸腺肽 a_1 及其他小分子多肽;辅料为氯化钠。
【性　　状】本品为无色或微黄色澄明液体。
【适 应 症】用于治疗各种原发性或继发性 T 细胞缺陷病,某些自身免疫性疾病,各种细胞免疫功能低下的疾病及肿瘤的辅助治疗。
【规　　格】5ml:40mg
【用法用量】皮下或肌内注射。一次 10~20mg,一日 1 次或遵医嘱。静脉滴注。一次 20~80mg,溶于 500ml0.9%氯化钠注射液或 5%葡萄糖注射液,一日 1 次或遵医嘱。
【不良反应】尚不明确。
【禁　　忌】阳性反应者禁用。
【注意事项】1、对于过敏体质者,注射前或治疗终止后再用药时需做皮内敏感试验(配成 25μg/ml 的溶液,皮内注射 0.1ml),阳性反应者禁用。2、本品如出现浑浊或絮状沉淀物等异常变化,禁止使用。
【孕妇及哺乳期妇女用药】尚不明确。
【儿童用药】尚不明确。
【老年用药】尚不明确。
【药物相互作用】尚不明确。
【药物过量】尚不明确。
【药理毒理】药理作用 药效学:本品为免疫调节药。具有调节和增强人体细胞免疫功能的作用,能促使 T-淋巴细胞成熟。毒理研究 尚不明确。
【药代动力学】尚不明确。
【贮　　藏】密闭,在凉暗处(避光并不超过 20℃)保存。
【包　　装】低硼硅玻璃安瓿,10 支/盒
【有 效 期】18 个月
【执行标准】国家药品监督管理局国家药品标准 WS1-XG-043-2000
【批准文号】国药准字 H20044074
【生产企业】企业名称:湖南一格制药有限公司
生产地址:湖南省湘潭市北二环路 1689 号
邮政编码:411100
电话号码:(0732)8289818
传真号码:(0732)8289819

Fig. 1. An example of pharmaceutical instruction.

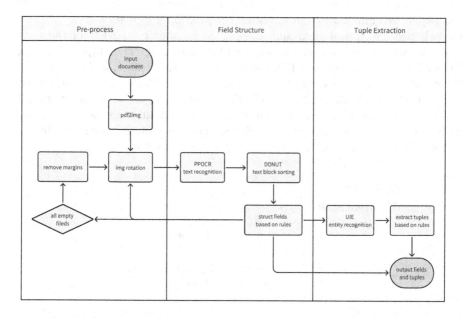

Fig. 2. The framework of the proposed model.

2.1   Preprocessing Module

In real-world situation, the pharmaceutical instructions we obtain are mainly in the form of images or PDF format data. To facilitate extraction with a unified method, we first convert PDFs into images. Secondly, different images can have problems with orientation. Therefore, we use a model to classify the orientation to determine whether the image needs to be rotated, including rotations of 0, 90, 180, and 270° as classification targets; Finally, images often contain large blank areas, which can adversely affect text recognition. Therefore, we use OpenCV [2] to identify large blank spaces in the image and then remove them from the image.

2.2   Textualization Module

To carry out information extraction, we first need to convert the image-format pharmaceutical instructions into a sequence of pure text format. We use PPOCR for text recognition, but the formats of pharmaceutical instruction manuals are varied, including single-column, double-column, and other different formats. PPOCR [4] cannot automatically concatenate the text boxes correctly after recognition, so we use DONUT for the correct concatenation of text recognition blocks. Specifically, we shuffle the sequence, and then use DONUT to input the serial number and the position of the text boxes. We train DONUT [3] with this data to output the correct sequence. This procedure is shown in Fig. 3. In this paper, we employ PPOCR to obtain the position information corresponding to each text block and then add a sequence number to the left of the position information, which is the result used for reordering. The output using the DONUT model is a sequence (63, 23, 45, 61, 62, 41, 52, 49, 5, 3, 44, 13, 58, 46, 22, 29, 60, 38, 10, 36, 14, 42, 43, 20, 57, 7, 34, 9, 37, 55, 54, 27, 18, 15, 50, 16, 39, 8 , 12, 25, 0, 6, 35, 26, 31, 21, 17, 47, 19, 59, 28, 1, 40, 4, 30, 53, 2, 24, 32, 56, 48), where the number corresponds to the serial number in the picture, and then the serial number is used to stitch together the contents recognized by the PPOCR to form a textual version of the pharmaceutical manual.

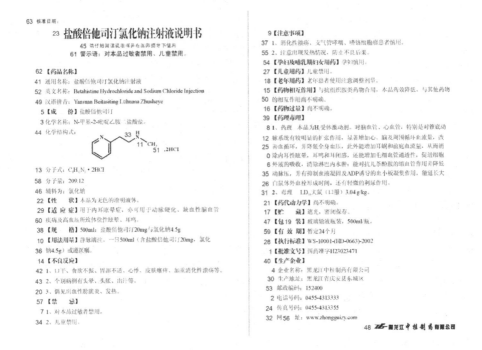

Fig. 3. The illustration of text chunks rearrangement.

2.3   Information Extraction Module

After completing the conversion of pharmaceutical instructions from image format to text format as described above, this paper carries out knowledge extraction based on these text data. Given the length of pharmaceutical instruction manuals and the different content described in each text section, such as indications, usage and dosage, contraindications, etc., Table 1 details the lengths of different text sections. To better carry out knowledge extraction, this paper first uses a rule-based method to divide the pharmaceutical instruction manuals into several different text blocks, each block describing a type of content, such as indications. On the entire textual content of the instruction manual, rule-based extraction is conducted to extract the content of 17 specified fields. On this basis, this paper uses UIE [5] for entity recognition. Given the limited training data provided for this evaluation task, this paper uses publicly available medical NER [1,9] data and some accumulated data for entity recognition. This step identifies the entities in the text blocks, such as diseases and symptom entities within the indications, dosage descriptions within the usage and dosage, etc. Different text blocks describe different attributes of the drug; therefore, this paper uses a rule-based method to concatenate the identified entities to construct triples, like all entities extracted from the indications block in the pharmaceutical instructions are the indications of the drug. For example, entities like "tumor" and "autoimmune disease" are extracted from the indications block shown in Fig. 1, and then triples such as (Thymosin Injection, Indications, Tumor) and (Thymosin Injection, Indications, Autoimmune Disease) can be constructed.

Table 1. The lengths of different text sections.

sections	mean	std	max
Indications	67	75	454
Usage and Dosage	123	194	2532
Contraindications	40	51	520
Pharmacology and Toxicology	231	276	1741
Ingredients	78	50	413
Specifications	11	20	297
Precautions	260	483	6657
Medication for Pregnant and Lactating Women	46	82	1006
Pharmacokinetic	155	255	2956
Drug Interactions	144	254	2036
Adverse Reactions	150	231	2137
Storage	12	7	43
Product Names	1	1	10
Common Names	7	2	18
Description	15	9	138
Pediatric Use	22	45	686
Geriatric Use	22	38	390

3 Experiments

To assess the performance of the proposed method, we conduct experiments on CHIP2023-Recognition and Entity Relationship Extraction of Paper-based Drug Description.

3.1   Dataset

This study conducted experiments using the dataset from CHIP2023-Recognition and Entity Relationship Extraction of Pharmaceutical Instruction task. The training set contains 495 pharmaceutical instructions, the validation set contains 88 pharmaceutical instructions, and the test set is not made public and is respectively divided into A-list and B-list[2].

3.2   Experimental Settings

In this study, we employ the t5-pegasus-chinese as the generative model for UIE, and the Chinese pre-trained PPOCR model[3].

The validation set was used to search for the optimal hyperparameters and the number of iterations. And we implement our method based on Pytorch[4]. The final main experimental configuration consisted of the T5 model, 50 epochs, a batch size of 8, a dropout rate of 0.3, a pad size of 32, a learning rate of 0.0005ß, the max length is 768, warmup steps is 300. All experiments were conducted on a GPU server with the following specifications: 2 AMD EPYC 7742 CPUs, 512GB DDR4 memory, and 8 Nvidia A100 80GB graphics cards.

In this paper, we utilize cer, average-cer, macro-f1 and score to evaluate the models. These metrics are calculated using Eq. 1, where ED is the edit distance [6], Predict is the predicted result, Value is the correct value, len is the length of the given string, TP represents the number of positive instances that are correctly predicted, TN represents the number of negative instances that are correctly predicted, FP represents the number of negative instances that are incorrectly predicted as positive, and FN represents the number of positive instances that are incorrectly predicted as negative. Macro-f1 is the weighted average of the F1-value of all classes. The score is the most important metric for this task, the higher the score, the better the performance of pharmaceutical Instruction extraction.

$$cer = ED(Predict, Value)/len(Value)$$

$$P = \frac{TP}{TP + FP}$$

$$R = \frac{TP}{TP + FN}$$

$$F1 = \frac{2 * P * R}{P + R} \quad (1)$$

$$macro - F1 = \frac{1}{N} \sum_{i=1}^{N} F1_i$$

$$score = 0.3 * (1 - average - cer) + 0.7 * macro - F1$$

---

[2] https://tianchi.aliyun.com/competition/entrance/532140.
[3] https://github.com/PaddlePaddle/PaddleOCR..
[4] https://pytorch.org/.

3.3   Results

Table 2. The performances of our proposed method on test set A list and B list.

Test set	score	average-cer	macro-f1
A	0.1398	0.5509	0.0072
B	0.28	0.54	0.21

Table 3. The top five results of B list.

Test set	score	average-cer	macro-f1
Our	0.28	0.54	0.21
Second	0.09	0.69	0.00
Third	0.07	0.81	0.01
Forth	0.02	0.94	0.00
Fifth	0.00	0.99	0.00

We conducted experiments on the CHIP2023-Recognition and Entity Relationship Extraction of Pharmaceutical Instruction task, and the results of our method are present in Table 2, the top five results of this task are presented in Table 3. From the experimental results, we can draw the following conclusions:

- From the results, the method proposed in this paper achieved the best performance and significantly outperformed other competing methods (0.28 vs 0.09);
- However, from the extraction results, the overall extraction performance still cannot achieve high accuracy for pharmaceutical specification extraction, which is mainly due to the poor quality of the input images, including a large amount of noise information such as watermarks and stamps;
- We also verified through extensive experiments that the pipeline-based method is difficult to tune and requires more labeling signals.

4   Conclusion

This article proposes a method for extracting information from pharmaceutical instructions that combines rules and deep learning. The method can extract corresponding knowledge from images and PDF-format pharmaceutical instructions, mainly including three modules: preprocessing, text recognition and alignment, and knowledge extraction. Experimental results show that the method can achieve good results in real-world scenarios. However, this method is essentially a pipeline method composed of multiple modules, making the overall optimization of the model very difficult. In the future, we expect to achieve end-to-end pharmaceutical information extraction through multimodal large-scale models.

References

1. An, B.: Construction and application of Chinese breast cancer knowledge graph based on multi-source heterogeneous data. Math. Biosci. Eng. **20**(4), 6776–6799 (2023)
2. Culjak, I., Abram, D., Pribanic, T., Dzapo, H., Cifrek, M.: A brief introduction to opencv. In: 2012 Proceedings of the 35th International Convention MIPRO, pp. 1725–1730. IEEE (2012)
3. Kim, G., et al.: Donut: document understanding transformer without OCR. arXiv preprint arXiv:2111.15664 7, 15 (2021)
4. Li, C., et al.: Pp-ocrv3: more attempts for the improvement of ultra lightweight OCR system. arXiv preprint arXiv:2206.03001 (2022)
5. Lu, Y., et al.: Unified structure generation for universal information extraction. arXiv preprint arXiv:2203.12277 (2022)
6. Ristad, E.S., Yianilos, P.N.: Learning string-edit distance. IEEE Trans. Pattern Anal. Mach. Intell. **20**(5), 522–532 (1998)
7. Thirunavukarasu, A.J., Ting, D.S.J., Elangovan, K., Gutierrez, L., Tan, T.F., Ting, D.S.W.: Large language models in medicine. Nat. Med. **29**(8), 1930–1940 (2023)
8. Wang, S., et al.: An interpretable data-driven medical knowledge discovery pipeline based on artificial intelligence. IEEE J. Biomed. Health Inform. (2023)
9. Yepes, A.J., MacKinlay, A.: NER for medical entities in twitter using sequence to sequence neural networks. In: Proceedings of the Australasian Language Technology Association Workshop 2016, pp. 138–142 (2016)
10. Zhongyong, C., Yongsheng, H., Min, Z., Ming, J.: A study on entity extraction method for pharmaceutical instructions based on pretrained models. J. Front. Comput. Sci. Technol. 1

CHIP-YIER Medical Large Model Evaluation

Overview of CHIP2023 Shared Task 4: CHIP-YIER Medical Large Language Model Evaluation

Han Hu[1], Jun Yan[2], Xiaozhen Zhang[2], Zengtao Jiao[2], and Buzhou Tang[1,3(✉)]

[1] Harbin Institute of Technology (Shenzhen), Shenzhen 518055, Guangdong, China
tangbuzhou@hit.edu.cn
[2] YiDu Tech, Beijing, China
{jun.yan,zengtao.jiao}@yiducloud.com
[3] Pengcheng Laboratory, Shenzhen 518055, Guangdong, China

Abstract. In recent years, large language models (LLMs) have demonstrated outstanding performance in natural language processing (NLP) tasks, showcasing remarkable capabilities in semantic understanding, text generation, and complex task reasoning. This emerging technology has also been applied to medical artificial intelligence, spanning traditional medical NLP tasks such as medical information extraction and medical entity normalization to practical applications in medical diagnosis, personalized treatment plan formulation, drug research and optimization, and early disease prediction. LLMs have achieved surprising results in these medical tasks. Major research institutions, universities, and companies have successively released their own large language models. However, due to the high risk characteristic of the medical industry, it is crucial to ensure their accuracy and reliability in clinical applications. To address this concern, the China Health Information Processing Conference (CHIP) introduced the evaluation task "CHIP-YIER Medical Large Model Evaluation" to assess the performance of large models in medical terminology, medical knowledge, adherence to clinical standards in diagnosis and treatment, and other medical aspects. The evaluation dataset is presented in the form of multiple-choice questions, comprising 1000 training set examples and 500 test set examples. Participating teams are required to select the correct answers based on the given descriptions. A total of 12 teams submitted valid results, with the highest F1 score of 0.7646.

Keywords: Medical · Large Language Model · Evaluation Metric

1 Introduction

Since the release of GPT-3 by OpenAI, LLMs have undergone continuous evolution, demonstrating superior performance across various NLP tasks [1]. In the field of biomedicine, artificial intelligence technology is experiencing a significant transition from traditional pre-trained language models (PLMs) to large language models (LLMs) [2]. The ongoing advancements and iterations in LLMs technology have successfully addressed numerous challenges in the field of medical artificial intelligence. The robust conversational and interactive capabilities of LLMs offer substantial support for online medical consultation systems, leading to a significant reduction in human resource costs. The Chain-of-Thought (CoT) method [3] guides LLMs in gradual thinking and reasoning, empowering them to analyze and address complex medical problems. Challenges such as the difficulty and high cost of annotating training data in the medical domain, along with concerns about patient privacy, have been mitigated through solutions like few-shot learning [4] and zero-shot learning [5].

Currently, LLMs have found practical applications in the medical field, encompassing medical image diagnosis, personalized treatment plan formulation, drug research and optimization, and early disease prediction [6–8]. However, the clinical application of LLMs still entails high risks, as errors, ambiguity, or incomplete information could potentially jeopardize patients' lives. Therefore, assessing the accuracy and reliability of LLMs is of paramount importance [9].

In response to this challenge, the 9th China Health Information Processing Conference (CHIP) focused on "Large Models and Intelligent Healthcare" and introduced six evaluation tasks, including the "CHIP-YIER Medical Large Language Model Evaluation" task. This evaluation task aims to assess LLMs through logical reasoning, examining their performance in medical terminology, medical knowledge, adherence to clinical standards in diagnosis and treatment, and other medical aspects within the context of the Chinese language. The results of this evaluation hold significant reference value for the clinical application of LLMs in China.

2 Related Work

2.1 Medical LLMs Evaluation Benchmarks

With the rapid development of medical LLMs, the comprehensive and accurate evaluation of their performance has become a crucial issue. In the English context, there are some authoritative evaluation tasks or datasets like I2B2/N2B2, USMLE, MedQA, PubMedQA [10], and MedMCQA [11]. Among these, I2B2/N2B2, initiated by the National Institutes of Health and the Biomedical Informatics Department at Harvard Medical School, consists of a series of evaluation tasks and workshops focusing on unstructured medical record data, gaining wide influence in the medical NLP community. USMLE comprises questions from the United States Medical Licensing Examination. MedQA encompasses multiple-choice questions collected from medical licensing exams in the United States, mainland China, and Taiwan. PubMedQA is the first question answering (QA) dataset derived from PubMed abstracts, containing 1,000 expert annotations, 61.2k unlabeled, and 211.3k artificially generated QA instances. MedMCQA consists of multiple-choice questions from simulated exams and past exams released by two medical schools in India.

In the Chinese context, Professor Wang Xiaoling's team from the School of Computer Science at East China Normal University, in collaboration with Alibaba Tianchi Platform, Fudan University, Fudan University-affiliated Huashan Hospital, Northeast University, Harbin Institute of Technology (Shenzhen), Peng Cheng Laboratory, and

Tongji University, introduced the PromptCBLUE evaluation benchmark. This benchmark transforms 16 different medical NLP tasks into prompt-based language generation tasks, forming the first Chinese medical LLMs evaluation benchmark. The Chinese University of Hong Kong (Shenzhen), in conjunction with the Shenzhen Big Data Research Institute, proposed the Comprehensive Medical Benchmark in Chinese (CMB) [12]. It includes multiple-choice questions from different clinical professions and different career stages (CMB-Exam) and complex clinical diagnostic problems based on real cases (CMB-Clin).

However, evaluating medical LLMs in Chinese still faces challenges. Firstly, there is a scarcity of authoritative evaluation datasets, and the existing datasets suffer from issues such as small scale, lack of comprehensiveness, and difficulties in replication. These challenges make it challenging to compare the performance of different models on a common and objective benchmark, thereby reducing the credibility of model evaluations [13]. Recognizing this, CHIP introduced the "CHIP-YIER Medical Large Model Evaluation" task with the aim of establishing a unified Chinese benchmark for the evaluation of LLMs. The results of the evaluation provide clear directions for the future optimization and iteration of LLMs, and have significant reference for the continued application of LLMs in clinical healthcare settings.

2.2 Related Techniques

Parameter-Efficient Tuning. The term "large" in LLMs refers to their massive parameter size. Faced with models having parameters in the order of hundreds of millions, both pre-training and full-fine-tuning methods incur substantial time and monetary costs, making it challenging for general institutions and organizations to provide support for such expenses. Consequently, various methods for parameter-efficient tuning have been proposed. These methods achieve parameter efficiency by either training only a subset of model parameters or by freezing pre-trained model parameters and training additional lightweight modules to reduce the parameter size.

For example, Microsoft Research introduced the LoRA framework [14], which leverages the intrinsic low-rank characteristics of LLMs by introducing bypass matrices to simulate full-parameter fine-tuning. Stanford University presented prefix-tuning [15], which adds a trainable embedding layer on top of the original model for filtering information by adding prefixes to prompt words. Google proposed prompt tuning [16], a simplified version of prefix-tuning that selects only a subset of existing parameters to create prefix prompts. Tsinghua University introduced p-tuning v2 [17], an improved version of prompt tuning that adds prefix prompts not only at the input layer but also at every layer of the pre-trained model, allowing information to propagate to deeper layers of the model.

Parameter-efficient tuning methods significantly reduce the required parameter size during training. With appropriate selected training parameters, this approach allows LLMs to better learn domain-specific knowledge, thereby adapting to downstream tasks more effectively. Consequently, in the era of LLMs, parameter-efficient tuning methods have become an indispensable technology.

Prompt Learning. The "pretrain+fine-tuning" training paradigm mentioned in the previous section, while reducing the training costs of the model, still demands a substantial amount of training data during the fine-tuning phase. In the medical field, manual data annotation is hard, expensive, and involves privacy concerns, making it extremely difficult to obtain a large volume of professionally accurate data. The "pretrain+prompt+predict" training paradigm [18] addresses this issue and significantly diminishes the amount of training data required compared to fine-tuning.

The method of prompt learning can be summarized as selecting a suitable prompt template and transforming the downstream task into natural language form to closely align with the learning samples of the pre-trained model. This way, the upstream pre-trained model can accomplish specific tasks with minimal data. The key to prompt learning lies in the design of the prompt template, and there are two main methods: manual design and automatic generation. Manual designation of templates is intuitive but requires the designer to have prior knowledge of the pre-trained model. Automatically generated templates can be discrete or continuous. Different prompt templates can have a significant impact on predictions. Therefore, choosing appropriate templates according to the pre-trained model and downstream tasks is both crucial and challenging.

3 Task Details

3.1 Task Description

In this task, the model must accurately comprehend and logically infer terms and knowledge in the medical domain. It should be capable of performing calculations and deductions based on medical formulas, precisely grasp patient symptoms, and provide appropriate clinical diagnostic knowledge. The data is presented in the form shown in Fig. 1, with each dataset containing six attributes: {*context, question, selection, answer_choices, sample_id, source*}. Figure 2 illustrates two samples. Participating teams need to design their own algorithms to enable LLMs to answer {*question*} based on the medical text content in the {*context*}. The candidate options for the questions are stored in the {*selection*} field. When submitting answers, teams need to insert the model's predicted answers into each test data, with the keyword "predict_answers" and the value being a list of correct answers. Finally, the Micro Average F1 value is used as the evaluation metric.

Data Format

"context": str,   *(refers to the medical text, ignore some questions without medical text)*

"question":str,   *(refers to the stem question)*

"selection": [str1, str2, str3, str4],   *(indicates the candidate text item)*

"answer_choices": [str2, str4],   *(the correct answer, one or more from "selection")*

"sample_id": str,   *(refers to the test number prepared by the evaluation team)*

"source": str   *(refers to the source of the question, such as the true question of practicing physicians, the true question of clinical tests, and the self-written question of medical experts)*

Fig. 1. Form of data

Sample: case 1

{

    "context": " （左侧前列腺）穿刺活检：腺癌（GLeason评分4+3=7分，分级分组3组），癌组织约占穿刺总体积70%。 （右侧前

列腺）穿刺活检：腺癌（GLeason评分4+4=8分，分级分组4组，），癌组织约占穿刺总体积60%。 ",

    "question": "从上述文本中结构化出的【肿瘤部位】正确的是（）",

    "selection": ["前列腺","卵巢","盆腔","腹部","以上都不对"],

    "answer_choices": ["前列腺"],

    "sample_id": "sample_13451",

    "source": "医学专家自拟题"

}

Sample: case 2

{

    "context": "",

    "question": "关于补体调控叙述正确的是",

    "selection": ["补体激活过程中生成的中间产物不稳定","只有结合在细胞表面的抗原抗体复合物才能触发经典途径","补体系统

活化失控可造成自身损伤"，"产生病理效应","细胞表面结合有多种补体调节因子","补体调节蛋白有十余种"],

    "answer_choices": ["补体激活过程中生成的中间产物不稳定","只有结合在细胞表面的抗原抗体复合物才能触发经典途径","补

体系统活化失控可造成自身损伤"，"细胞表面结合有多种补体调节因子"],

    "sample_id": "sample_1",

    "source": "临床考研真题"

}

Fig. 2. Data samples

3.2 Dataset

The evaluation data is constructed based on real clinical scenarios, including a series of multiple-choice questions derived from medical postgraduate entrance exams, clinical practice questions for licensed physicians, medical textbooks, medical literature/guidelines, and publicly available medical case records. The dataset is divided into training and testing sets to ensure the model's generalization across different data distributions. The evaluation data is released in two phases. The training set, comprising 1000 datas, was released on September 10, 2023. The testing set consists of 500 datas, with the {*answer_choices*} field left empty, and was released on September 25, 2023.

3.3 Evaluation Metric

The answers in the dataset are multiple-choice, so this evaluation employs the Micro Average F1 score as the evaluation metric. By summing the quantities of True Positives (TP), False Positives (FP), and False Negatives (FN) for all answers, the overall Precision, Recall, and F1 Score are calculated according to formulas (1)–(3).

$$Precision = \frac{TP}{TP + FP} \tag{1}$$

$$Recall = \frac{TP}{TP + FN} \tag{2}$$

$$F1 = 2 \times \frac{Precision \times Recall}{Precision + Recall} \tag{3}$$

4 Submission Result

4.1 Overall Statistics

As of the submission deadline, there are a total of 15 participating teams, with 12 teams submitting their final answers. The statistical results are presented in Table 1.

Table 1. Overall statistical result of CHIP2023 shared task4.

Metric	max	min	average	median	std
Precision	0.7699	0.12	0.3778	0.3549	0.1677
Recall	0.7594	0.1024	0.3487	0.3055	0.1629
F1 Score	0.7646	0.1105	0.3621	0.3297	0.1647

4.2 Top Two Models

Table 2 shows the scores of the top two models in this task. And we will give a brief introduction to their models.

Table 2. Scores of the top two models.

Ranking	Precision	Recall	F1 Score
1st	0.7699	0.7594	0.7646
2nd	0.582	0.5085	0.5428

The first team proposes a framework based on ChatGPT fusion ensemble learning to achieve question answering in the medical domain. The method can be divided into three steps. In the first step, they design some prompt templates and let ChatGPT play the role of a professional clinical expert or an AI-assisted doctor to obtain multiple results. The second step involves regular expression processing. Answers generated by the large language models may contain explanatory language, so they need to extract the specific answers within square brackets "[]". In the last step, they adopt the simplest ensemble learning method of majority voting to select one from multiple answers as their prediction result. They run the training dataset on HuatuoGPT and ChatGPT and observe that ChatGPT performs better, so they decide to use ChatGPT for prediction.

The method proposed by the second team also consists of three steps. In the first step, they employ the date argument method and utilize an additional MATH dataset to enhance the computational ability of the model. For data augmentation, they design several prompt templates based on the {*context*}, {*question*}, and {*answer_choices*} in the dataset to guide ChatGLM in generating explanations for answers. Subsequently, multiple explanations are sent to ChatGPT, which assigns scores to them. The explanation with the highest score is selected as the final training sample. In the training step, they use ChatGLM2-6B as the base model and fine-tune it with the QLoRA framework. To adjust the parameters, they divide the training and validation sets in the ratio of 7:3. In the inference step, they use the Chain-of-Thought method to guide the fine-tuned model in generating answers.

5 Conclusion

This article introduces the details of the CHIP2023 evaluation task4 "CHIP-YIER Medical Large Language Model Evaluation", including international and domestic benchmarks for LLMs evaluation, parameters-efficient tuning, prompt learning, overall participation in this evaluation, and the model approaches of two outstanding teams. The first team chose ChatGPT as the evaluation model, employing prompt learning and ensemble learning techniques. The second team selected ChatGLM2-6B as the baseline model, fine-tuned it using the QLoRA framework, and combined data augmentation with prompt learning techniques. The evaluation results indicate that there is still room for improvement in the performance of LLMs in the medical domain. It is recommended to conduct ongoing evaluation tasks to establish a unified, comprehensive, and refined evaluation system for LLMs. This will serve as an important reference for the application of LLMs in the healthcare industry.

Acknowledgments. This study is partially supported by National Key RD Program of China (2021ZD0113402), National Natural Science Foundation of China (62276082), Major Key Project of PCL (PCL2021A06), Shenzhen Soft Science Research Program Project (RKX20220705152815035) and the Fundamental Research Fund for the Central Universities (HIT.DZJJ.2023117).

References

1. Mao, R., Chen, G., Zhang, X., et al.: GPTEval: a survey on assessments of ChatGPT and GPT-4. J. CoRR abs/2308.12488 (2023)
2. He, K., Mao, R., Lin, Q., et al.: A survey of large language models for healthcare: from data, technology, and applications to accountability and ethics. J. arXiv preprint arXiv:2310.05694 (2023)
3. Wei, J., Wang, X., Schuurmans, D., et al.: Chain-of-thought prompting elicits reasoning in large language models. J. Adv. Neural Inf. Process. Syst. **35**, 24824–24837 (2022)
4. Ma, Y., Wang, Z., Cao, Y., et al.: Few-shot event detection: an empirical study and a unified view. J. arXiv preprint arXiv:2305.01901 (2023)
5. Hu, Y., Ameer, I., Zuo, X., et al.: Zero-shot clinical entity recognition using ChatGPT. J. CoRR abs/2303.16416 (2023)
6. Alhaidry, H.M., Fatani, B., Alrayes, J.O., et al.: ChatGPT in dentistry: a comprehensive review. J. Cureus. **15**, e38317 (2023)
7. Srivastav, S., Chandrakar, R., Gupta, S., et al.: ChatGPT in radiology: the advantages and limitations of artificial intelligence for medical imaging diagnosis. J. Cureus, 15(7) (2023)

8. Cheng, K., Li, Z., He, Y., et al.: Potential use of artificial intelligence in infectious disease: take ChatGPT as an example. J. Ann. Biomed. Eng. 1–6 (2023)

9. Jin, Y., Chandra, M., Verma, G., et al.: Better to ask in english: cross-lingual evaluation of large language models for healthcare queries. J. arXiv e-prints, arXiv: 2310.13132 (2023)

10. Jin, Q., Dhingra, B., Liu, Z., et al.: Pubmedqa: a dataset for biomedical research question answering. J. arXiv preprint arXiv:1909.06146 (2019)

11. Pal, A., Umapathi, L.K., Sankarasubbu, M.: Medmcqa: a large-scale multi-subject multi-choice dataset for medical domain question answering. In: Conference on Health, Inference, and Learning. pp. 248–260. PMLR (2022)

12. Wang, X., Chen, G.H., Song, D., et al.: Cmb: a comprehensive medical benchmark in Chinese. J. arXiv preprint arXiv:2308.08833 (2023)

13. 颜见智, 何雨鑫, 骆子烨, 等. 生成式大语言模型在医疗领域的潜在典型应用与面临的挑战. J. 医学信息学杂志, 44(09):23–31 (2023)

14. Hu, E.J., Shen, Y., Wallis, P., et al.: Lora: low-rank adaptation of large language models. J. arXiv preprint arXiv:2106.09685 (2021)

15. Li, X.L., Liang, P.: Prefix-tuning: optimizing continuous prompts for generation. J. arXiv preprint arXiv:2101.00190 (2021)

16. Lester, B., Al-Rfou, R., Constant, N.: The power of scale for parameter-efficient prompt tuning. J. arXiv preprint arXiv:2104.08691 (2021)

17. Liu, X., Ji, K., Fu, Y., et al.: P-tuning v2: prompt tuning can be comparable to fine-tuning universally across scales and tasks. J. arXiv preprint arXiv:2110.07602 (2021)

18. Liu, P., Yuan, W., Fu, J., et al.: Pre-train, prompt, and predict: a systematic survey of prompting methods in natural language processing. J. ACM Comput. Surv. **55**(9), 1–35 (2023)

A Medical Diagnostic Assistant Based on LLM

Chengyan Wu[1], Zehong Lin[1], Wenlong Fang[1], and Yuyan Huang[1,2(✉)]

[1] School of Electronics and Information Engineering,
South China Normal University, Foshan 528225, China
{chengyan.wu,linzehong,20153100003}@m.scnu.edu.cn
[2] Datastory, Guangzhou, China
yuyan@datastory.com.cn

Abstract. With the advent of ChatGPT, large language models (LLMs) have received extensive attention because of their excellent instruction comprehension and generation capabilities. However, LLMs are not specifically designed for the healthcare domain and still lack accuracy in answering specialized healthcare-related questions. In this paper, we mainly used some approaches to improve the performance of large language models in the medical domain. First, we analyzed and processed data to ensure high quality and consistency. Second, we used the model's excellent ability to generate inference process to the training data. Finally, the data with the explanation and inference process, which are helpful in guiding the thinking and improving the inference ability of the model, are used for training. In terms of model training, we used ChatGLM2-6B as the base model, and the large language model was fine-tuned using the QLoRA framework. To guide the model to generate compliant outputs better, we also explored and carefully constructed appropriate prompts. Overall, our approachs enable the model to achieve the F1 value of 0.433 in this task.

Keywords: Medical question answering · Large language models · Data augmentation · Chain of thought · Instruction fine-tuning

1 Introduction

Since the emergence of ChatGPT, large language models (LLMs) have received widespread attention because of their excellent command comprehension and generation capabilities. Compared with previous smaller language models, large language models are trained using large amounts of textual data, thereby showing strong generalization capabilities on many NLP tasks and in solving unknown or complex tasks.

The application of LLMs in clinical diagnosis and medical research is a promising area, where they can help doctors and patients to improve the efficiency and quality of diagnosis, treatment, and prevention. They can also help

---

C. Wu, Z. Lin and W. Fang—These authors contributed equally to this work.

H. Xu et al. (Eds.): CHIP 2023, CCIS 2080, pp. 135–147, 2024.
https://doi.org/10.1007/978-981-97-1717-0_12

medical researchers to discover new knowledge and methods. Despite the many advantages of LLMs, they are not specifically designed for the medical field and lack accuracy in answering some specialized questions related to healthcare. The medical field has a very low tolerance for error and a very high compliance requirement. Hence, accuracy and reliability are crucial in this field. In response to the aforementioned problems, several LLMs, such as MedPaLM, HuatuoGPT [1], and DoctorGLM [2], have been developed specifically for healthcare vertical applications. The application of these medical LLMs has become an important tool for improving patient care and diagnosis. The 9th Chinese Health Information Processing Conference (CHIP2023) focuses on "Large Language Models and Intelligent Healthcare" and gathers top medical information processing scholars and medical experts to discuss the trends and challenges of the development of intelligent healthcare in the context of the era of LLMs, new paths of AI medical applications, and new methods of medical research. Six evaluation tasks are organized for this conference, among which, Task 4 is the Medical LLM Evaluation Task, which aims to examine the performance of the medical LLMs in medical aspects, such as medical terminology, medical knowledge, clinical specification diagnosis and treatment, and medical computation through the evaluation of the logical reasoning. In this task, the model needs to understand and logically explain medical terminologies, medical knowledge, clinical standardized diagnosis and treatment, and medical computations. The main tasks cover the following aspects: the model needs to accurately understand and logically deduce medical terminology and knowledge; the model must be able to perform calculations and derivations based on medical formulas, accurately grasp the patient's symptoms, and provide appropriate and specialized clinical diagnosis and treatment knowledge.

In this paper, we developed a solution based on the evaluation dataset provided by the organizer according to the characteristics of the task and the advantages of the LLM. We first analyzed and processed the data to ensure high quality and consistency. In addition, we adopted a data enhancement approach, using the model's own reasoning ability to supplement the training data by explanations based on the answers in the training data, and then training the model with the data from the interpreting and reasoning process, which is conducive to guiding the model's thinking and improving its reasoning ability. For model training, we adopt ChatGLM2-6B as the base model, use the QLora framework to fine-tune the larger model, and select appropriate parameters based on the model's performance in the validation set to enable the model to better adapt to the evaluation task. We also explored and carefully constructed appropriate prompts to guide the model in generating compliant outputs.

The main contributions of this work are as follows:

- We process and augment data. By making full use of the capabilities of the model, we use data augmentation while constructing answers according to the Chain-of-Thought (CoT)'s data format, thereby guiding the model into deeper thinking.

- We adopt ChatGLM2-6B as the base model and make supervised instruction fine-tuning with the help of the QLoRA framework to enhance the model's reasoning capabilities. This step aims at better adapting the model to the needs of a specific task and improving its accuracy and efficiency in the reasoning process.
- We explored and construct prompts. By finding prompt templates suitable for a particular task as input to the model, we guided the model to output answers that meet the requirements. This step aims to optimize input information to guide the model more efficiently in generating suitable output.

2 Related Work

2.1 LLMs for Medication

In recent years, LLMs have made considerable progress in the field of AI. LLMs, such as GPT-3 [3], LLaMA [4], and PaLM [5], have demonstrated impressive capabilities in a wide range of natural language tasks. Despite the excellent performance of these models, OpenAI has yet to reveal details of their training strategies or weighting parameters. Although LLaMA is an open source, its results on Chinese tasks are poor because its training data are mainly based on the English corpus. To solve the problem of LLMs on Chinese-specific task applications, Du et al. [6] proposed GLM, an autoregressive pre-training model with 130 billion parameters and multiple training objectives. Zeng et al. [7] proposed ChatGLM-6B based on the GLM architecture, which is a 6.2 billion-parameter bilingual Chinese-English support and open-source dialog language model. ChatGLM2-6B, the base model used in this paper, is an upgraded version of the first-generation model with higher performance, longer context, and more efficient inference.

Although LLMs perform well in general domains, they do not perform well in domains that require expertise (e.g., biomedical) because they lack domain-specific knowledge. To address this problem, many LLMs in the medical domain have been created. MedPaLM [8] is a variant of PaLM [5] that aims to provide high-quality answers to medical questions using command-prompt tuning techniques. ChatDoctor [9] is the first model that fine-tune LLaMa [4] using a general-purpose dataset and a doctor-patient dialog dataset to better understand the patient's needs and to provide recommendations. DoctorGLM [2] is a Chinese medical LLM trained using a Chinese medical dialog database derived from the ChatDoctor [9] dataset and translated using the ChatGPT API. In addition, it employs LoRA [10] technology, which reduces inference time. BenTsao [11] is a LLaMA-based LLM that has been supervised-fine-tuned using generated QA instances. The model was trained using structured and unstructured medical knowledge to ensure factual accuracy in its responses. Overall, these works highlight the potential for the successful application of LLMs in the medical domain.

2.2 Question Answering Task in Medication

The traditional question-and-answer (QA) task is a stand-alone task that is primarily designed to generate or retrieve appropriate answers based on the question posed. In the healthcare domain, QA systems have substantial benefits for healthcare professionals to locate necessary information in clinical records or literature, as well as to provide basic healthcare knowledge to patients. A robust healthcare quality assurance system can go a long way in meeting the counselling needs of patients. Many studies have explored the adaption of a generic pre-trained language model (PLM) to answer healthcare questions. For example, Pergola et al. [12] proposed an entity-aware masking strategy to ensure biomedical quality under low-resource conditions; Lee et al. [13] proposed BioBERT, a pre-trained biomedical language representation model for biomedical text mining; and Chen et al. [14] proposed the introduction of an external healthcare knowledgebase to augment medical visual and linguistic pre-training. However, it is difficult for PLM-based QA systems to play an essential role in real-world healthcare scenarios because of the presence of limited language comprehension and generation capabilities. With the advent of powerful LLMs, prompt-based approaches have been introduced to address QA tasks in the medical domain. The application of medical LLMs has become an important tool for improving patient care and diagnosis. Considering the uncertainty of answers generated by LLMs, ensuring the accuracy and reliability of these models becomes crucial in clinical applications. To assess the accuracy, relevance, comprehensiveness, and coherence of answers generated by LLMs, many scholars have made great efforts. For example, Ankit Pal et al. [15] proposed MedMCQA, a multiple-choice question dataset for medical entrance exams; Qiao Jin et al. [16] proposed Pub-MedQA dataset for answering yes/no/maybe based on the question summaries; and Dan Hendrycks et al. [17] proposed MMLU, a new test dataset for measuring the multitasking accuracy of text models.

In this CHIP-YIER Medical Large Language Models evaluation task, the organizers constructed a series of multiple-choice questions based on real clinical situations, which were used to test the performance of the LLMs in medical knowledge, clinically standardized diagnosis and treatment, and medical computation and other medical aspects.

2.3 Chain-of-Thought

Chain-of-Thought (CoT), first proposed by Wei et al. [18], is a prompting technology guide the LLMs to generate intermediate reasoning steps that lead to the final answer. Some recent studies have demonstrated that thought chains can remarkably improve model capabilities. Zhou et al. [19] propose least-to-most prompting, a novel prompting strategy that decomposes a complex problem into a series of simpler sub-problems and then solved them sequentially. Zhang et al. [20] proposed AutoCoT, an automatic CoT prompting method that sampled questions with diversity and generated reasoning chains to build demonstrations. Additionally, in the zero-shot scenario, Kojima et al. [21] added some magic phrases to LLMs (e.g., "let's think in one step") to enable LLMs to generate proper intermediate steps. Zelikman et al. [22] used LLM to generate many intermediate steps and select the ones that might lead to the final answer. These studies show that CoT plays an important role in improving the reasoning ability of LLMs. Therefore, we also adopt the idea of CoT when designing solutions for the evaluation task.

2.4   Parameters-Efficient Optimizations

As LLMs become larger in terms of parameter size, fully fine-tuning the downstream task dataset becomes increasingly costly. To alleviate this problem, a series of parameter-efficient tuning methods have been proposed to help pretrained LLMs efficiently adapt to various downstream tasks. Usually, three typical approaches can be applied in efficient parameter optimization: adapter, prefix tuning, and LoRA. Adapter methods mainly add a new network module adapter inside the pre-trained model to adapt to the downstream tasks. Moreover, during the fine-tuning process, only the parameters of the adapter module are trained while keeping the rest of the model parameters fixed. Hu et al. [23] proposed LLM-Adapters, an easy-to-use framework for integrating various adapters into LLMs, which could be used to perform different tasks using these adapter-based PEFT methods for LLMs. Prefix tuning refers to the addition of a continuous sequence of task-specific learnable prefixes in front of model inputs or hidden layers. Taking inspiration from prompting, Li et al. [24] proposed the prefix tuning method, which enabled the use of large pre-trained language models by optimising a small continuous task-specific vector. Hu et al. [10] proposed the LoRA framework, the core of which was to use low-rank matrices to approximate the parameter updates of full-rank weight matrices, so that only a small ascending matrix and a small descending matrix need to be trained. In this paper, we use the QLoRA method [25], which is a low-precision quantization and fine-tuning technique for deep neural networks that enabled high-fidelity 4-bit fine-tuning, for efficient parameter tuning. The method uses a novel high-precision technique to quantize a pre-trained model to 4-bits and then adds a set of learnable low-rank adapter weights (low-rank adapter weights), which are tuned by backpropagating the gradients of the quantization weights.

3   Methodology

3.1   Model Structure

This section describes the framework designed for the medical LLM evaluation task. The overall framework is shown in Fig. 1 and is divided into three key parts: data processing and augmentation, model fine-tuning, and inference process. In the data processing and augmentation section, the raw data are initially processed and converted into a multiple-choice format that the model is good at handling. Then, reasoning content is added to the training data through three stages of manipulation to achieve the goal of data augmentation. In the model fine-tuning section, we selected ChatGLM2-6B as the base model and used the QLoRA framework for supervised instruction fine- tuning. This step aims to better adapt the model to specific tasks in the medical domain. During the model inference process, questions and prompt templates are cleverly spliced together and used as inputs to the model inference. Based on the input questions and choices, the model accurately selects the correct answers and generates the corresponding explanations. Finally, we use regular expressions to extract the specifics of the answers.

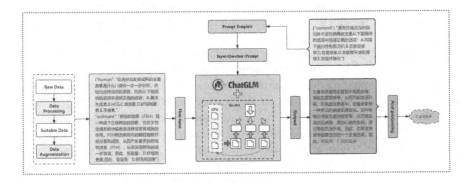

Fig. 1. Overview of model fine-tuning and inference pipeline.

3.2   Task Description

In the medical LLM evaluation task, models need to understand and logically explain medical terminologies, medical knowledge, clinical standard diagnosis and treatment, and medical calculations. The input to the model includes a given question and the corresponding answer options, and the goal of the model is to select one or more correct answers from these answer options to complete the answer to the question. Specifically, the input format of the task is $I = \{question, selections\}$, and the output format should be generated based on the question and the selected answer, in the form $O = \{answer\_choices\}$.

3.3   Data Augmentation

During the testing process, the results of model training directly using the dataset provided by the organizer were unsatisfactory mainly because the dataset in this evaluation task covers the fields of medical terminology, medical knowledge, clinical specification diagnosis and treatment, as well as medical computation, which requires the model to have excellent comprehension and logical reasoning abilities. To enhance the model's ability in medical understanding and reasoning, we used ChatGLM2-6B to perform data augmentation on the training data to add more reasoning content. The data augmentation process can be divided into three key stages, as shown in Fig. 2: generating explanation; scoring candidate response; and splicing question, response, and answer. The implementation of this series of stages is intended to enable the model to understand medical information more fully and to improve its reasoning ability in the face of complex medical problems.

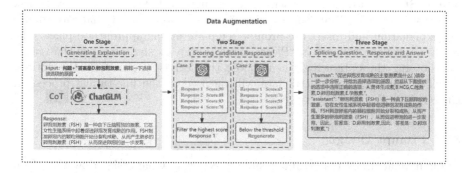

Fig. 2. Three stages of data augmentation.

One Stage: Generating Explanation. In this stage, we take the approach of transforming the questions from the training data into the form of multiple-choice questions, aligning them with the corresponding answers, and subsequently splicing them with a fixed prompt template. Ultimately, the form of the prompt is used as an input to the ChatGLM. By using such prompt template, we guide the model to think step-by-step based on the question and corresponding answer, thereby outputting explanations with a reasoning process.

Specifically, suppose $[x_i, y_i]^N$ denotes a dataset of N instances, where x_i is a question and y_i is the corresponding answer, and the prompt template e_i used is "The answer is: y_i, why? Please explain". The final prompt input to the LLMs is x_i, y_i, e_i, and the model will output an explanation of the corresponding answer to the question based on this input. This process will be repeated several times, resulting in multiple candidate explanations. In this way, we can guide the model to reason in a structured way, gradually going behind the questions and answers to generate more nuanced and logical explanations for the answer.

Two Stage: Scoring Candidate Response. Given that the unfine-tuned ChatGLM2-6B was used to generate explanations and reasoning processes for the answers, the content generated by the model was variable, and assessing the quality of the generated explanations became necessary. This step mainly involves scoring several candidate explanations generated in the first stage to filter out the explanation that is compatible with the answer.

In this evaluation process, we adopt ChatGPT as the scoring model. We used ChatGPT's API to score several candidate explanations and selected the explanation with the highest score that fits the question and the answer closely (Case

1). In addition, we set a scoring threshold, and when the scores of all candidate explanations generated by the ChatGLM are less than the set threshold (Case 2), then return to the previous step to regenerate explanations. Through this scoring process, we can effectively filter out explanations that are of high quality and consistent with the answers, thereby improving the overall accuracy and consistency of the explanations.

Three Stage: Splicing Question, Response and Answer. The main task at this stage is to skillfully splice together the question, answer, and corresponding explanation and insert the prompt template at the appropriate place. The prompt template we used is "Please think it step by step and give the reason for choosing the option and then choose the correct option from the options provided below". The spliced data will be used in the fine-tuning process of ChatGLM2-6B.

3.4   Prompt Design

LLMs have achieved remarkable results in conversational tasks. However, given that their output content can be unreliable and deceptive, we have added prompt to the input to improve the accuracy and reliability of the output. Different prompt templates have been explored and designed to suit different processes and objectives.

During "Generating Explanation", we used the following prompt template: "question" answer is "answer_choices", why? Please explain. For the test set, we used the following prompt template: "question" Please analyse step by step and give the reason for choosing the option and then choose the correct option from the options provided below: "selection". Here "question" denotes the question, "answer_choices" denotes the correct answer options and "selection" denotes the list of options. By testing these prompt templates, we found that they were effective in guiding the model to output the correct content and achieved a substantial improvement in effectiveness compared with the approach without prompt templates. This finding indicates that prompt templates play a key role in improving the quality of LLMs' output, helping to standardize and guide the model generation process.

3.5   Training of Our Model

ChatGLM2-6B is the selected base model. The full parameter fine-tuning of this model takes up considerable memory and time. To address this problem, we used an efficient fine-tuning method, QLoRA, for partial parameter fine-tuning. The method employs an innovative high-precision technique that quantizes the pretrained model to 4 bits and subsequently adds a set of learnable low-rank adapter weights. These weights are tuned by backpropagating the gradient of the quantized weights. Our trained data was augmented with explanations generated by large models. To enhance the computational power of the model, we also introduced a computational dataset (e.g., math dataset) for general domains. During the training process, we divided the training and validation sets in the ratio of 7:3, and continuously adjusted the model parameters based on the model's effect on the validation set. A total of 8 epochs of training were performed, with the learning rate set of 2×10^{-4} and batch_size of 12. The parameters used in QLoRA are detailed as follows: rank of 64, alpha of 16, and dropout of 0.05. These parameters were carefully tuned to ensure that the model achieves the best possible training performance.

3.6   Inference Process

After fine-tuning the aforementioned models, we used the trained ChatGLM2-6B model for inferring the questions in the test set. To guide the ChatGLM2-6B model in generating sensible responses relevant to the questions, a suitable prompt template must be constructed. The template could be in the form of, "Please analyze step-by-step and give reasons for choosing this option and then select the correct option from the options provided below". Such prompts help in guiding the model in generating structured and explanatory responses. The processed questions are spliced together with the prompt templates to form a sequence of inputs, and the splices are fed into the ChatGLM2-6B model to obtain the model's answers to the questions. Finally, considering that the result only needs to obtain to the answer without the associated reasoning process, we extract the answer options from the model-generated output via regular expressions to ensure that the extracted information conforms to the expected format and structure.

4   Experiments

4.1   Data Analysis

The assessment data are constructed based on actual clinical situations, including a series of multiple-choice questions constructed from medical examination questions, clinical practitioner questions, medical textbooks, medical literature/guidelines, and open medical records. The dataset contains diverse factors, such as different diseases, severity of conditions, and patient characteristics, to ensure the comprehensiveness and authenticity of the assessment. The dataset will be divided into a training set with 1000 pieces of data and a test set with 500 pieces of data, where the answer_choice field is empty. In addition, considering that the task involves the computation and derivation of medical formulas, we use an additional MATH dataset to fine-tune and improve the computational power of the model. The raw data provided by the organizer are tabulated in Table 1, where the number of single choice and multiple-choice questions in the training set are 905 and 95, respectively. During training, the training and validation sets are divided into a ratio of 7:3. Train# and Val# represent the training and validation sets, divided from the original training set, respectively.

Table 1. Quantitative analysis of raw data.

Type	Single-choice Question	Multiple-choice Question
Train	905	95
Train#	630	70
Val#	275	25

4.2 Parameter Settings

During the training process, we used the QLoRA framework to partially tune the parameters of the ChatGLM2-6B model for 8 epochs of training. The learning rate was set to 2×10^{-4} and the batch_size was 12. In addition, the parameters used by QLoRA in the fine-tuning included the QLoRA_rank Of 64, the QLoRA_alpha of 16, and the QLoRA_dropout of 0.05. The parameters of the specific model are listed in Table 2.

Table 2. Experimental parameter settings.

ChatGLM2-6B+ QLoRA	learning rate	2×10^{-4}
	epoch	8
	batch_size	12
	QLoRA_rank	64
	QLoRA_alpha	16
	QLoRA_dropout	0.05

4.3 Evaluation Indicators

Given that the answers in the dataset are obtained from multi-choice questions, the micro average F1 value is used as the evaluation metric. The overall precision, recall, and F1-Score are calculated by summing the number of true, false positive, and false negative cases for all answers.

$$\text{Micro Average Precision} = \frac{\text{Total Number of Correct Answers}}{\text{Total Number of Answers Recalled by Model}} \quad (1)$$

$$\text{Micro Average Recall} = \frac{\text{Total Correct Answers}}{\text{Total Answers in Test Data}} \quad (2)$$

$$\text{Micro Average F1} = \frac{2 \times (\text{Micro Average Precision} \times \text{Micro Average Recall})}{\text{Micro Average Precision} + \text{Micro Average Recall}} \quad (3)$$

4.4   Results

Table 3. The performance comparison between data augmentation and fine-tuning.

Method	Data	Precision	Recall	F1
ChatGLM2-6B+QLoRA+DA	Test	**0.449**	**0.418**	**0.433**
ChatGLM2-6B+QLoRA+DA	Val	**0.43**	**0.38**	**0.391**
ChatGLM2-6B+DA	Val	0.39	0.355	0.374
ChatGLM2-6B	Val	0.38	0.34	0.36

Table 3 shows the performance comparison between models using data augmentation and fine-tuning. As shown in the table, the model with data augmentation is superior in terms of precision, recall, and F1 in the split validation set compared with the model without additional data, thereby proving that a larger positive ground boost is obtained by expanding the common data for the same class of tasks. Specifically, the model with additional data achieves 39%, 35.5%, and 37.4% Precision, Recall, and F1 values on the validation set, respectively. Furthermore, the following observations, based on data augmentation, the model with efficient fine-tuning outperforms the results without fine-tuning in all three metrics, specifically, the model with efficient fine-tuning achieves 44.9%, 41.8%, and 43.3% Precision, Recall, and F1 values on the test set, respectively. The main reasons are detailed as follows: 1) Data augmentation adds an inference process to the training data, which can guide the model to think step-by-step and improve the accuracy and reliability of the inference. In addition, the introduction of common mathematical computation dataset can allow the model to adapt to some simple topics on medical computation, which enables the model to improve its computational ability. 2) Using efficient fine-tuning, the model can remarkably learn and adapt the features of a specific task. 3) The use of a combination of the two methods not only helps the model to improve its comprehensive ability but also use fewer resources to learn domain-specific features for specific downstream tasks.

5   Conclusion

In this paper, we propose a new framework aimed at improving the logical reasoning ability of LLMs, covering three phases, namely, data augmentation, fine-tuning, and inference. Specifically, the data enhancement phase uses the large-scale model to generate contents that contain thought processes for the training data. Then, an external tool, ChatGPT, sorts the candidate thought chains generated by the model multiple times, selects the optimal candidate answers, and splices them into replies. The augmented data are used to fine-tune the partial parameters in the fine-tuning phase, and the inference process involves reasoning about the questions in the test set to obtain answers. The experimental results show that the framework performs well and achieves high accuracy in the domains of medical terminology, medical knowledge, clinical standardized diagnosis and treatment, and medical computing. Finally, our model ranks second in the test set evaluation in the YIER Medical LLM evaluation task of CHIP 2023.

References

1. Zhang, H., et al.: HuatuoGPT, towards taming language model to be a doctor. arXiv preprint arXiv:2305.15075 (2023)
2. Xiong, H., et al.: DoctorGLM: fine-tuning your Chinese doctor is not a herculean task. arXiv preprint arXiv:2304.01097 (2023)
3. Brown, T., et al.: Language models are few-shot learners. In: Advances in Neural Information Processing Systems, vol. 33, pp. 1877–1901 (2020)
4. Touvron, H., et al.: LLaMA: open and efficient foundation language models. arXiv preprint arXiv:2302.13971 (2023)
5. Chowdhery, A., et al.: PaLM: scaling language modeling with pathways. arXiv preprint arXiv:2204.02311 (2022)
6. Du, Z., et al.: GLM: general language model pretraining with autoregressive blank infilling. arXiv preprint arXiv:2103.10360 (2021)
7. Zeng, A., et al.: GLM-130B: an open bilingual pre-trained model. arXiv preprint arXiv:2210.02414 (2022)
8. Singhal, K., et al.: Towards expert-level medical question answering with large language models. arXiv preprint arXiv:2305.09617 (2023)
9. Li, Y., Li, Z., Zhang, K., Dan, R., Zhang, Y.: ChatDoctor: a medical chat model fine-tuned on llama model using medical domain knowledge. arXiv preprint arXiv:2303.14070 (2023)
10. Hu, E.J., et al.: LoRA: low-rank adaptation of large language models. arXiv preprint arXiv:2106.09685 (2021)
11. Wang, H., et al.: HuaTuo: tuning llama model with Chinese medical knowledge. arXiv preprint arXiv:2304.06975 (2023)
12. Pergola, G., Kochkina, E., Gui, L., Liakata, M., He, Y.: Boosting low-resource biomedical QA via entity-aware masking strategies. arXiv preprint arXiv:2102.08366 (2021)
13. Lee, J., et al.: BioBERT: a pre-trained biomedical language representation model for biomedical text mining. Bioinformatics 36(4), 1234–1240 (2020)
14. Chen, Z., Li, G., Wan, X.: Align, reason and learn: enhancing medical vision-and-language pre-training with knowledge. In: Proceedings of the 30th ACM International Conference on Multimedia, pp. 5152–5161 (2022)
15. Pal, A., Umapathi, L.K., Sankarasubbu, M.: MedMCQA: a large-scale multi-subject multi-choice dataset for medical domain question answering. In: Conference on Health, Inference, and Learning, pp. 248–260. PMLR (2022)
16. Jin, Q., Dhingra, B., Liu, Z., Cohen, W.M., Lu, X.: PubMedQA: a dataset for biomedical research question answering. arXiv preprint arXiv:1909.06146 (2019)
17. Hendrycks, D., et al.: Measuring massive multitask language understanding. arXiv preprint arXiv:2009.03300 (2020)
18. Wei, J., et al.: Chain-of-thought prompting elicits reasoning in large language models. In: Advances in Neural Information Processing Systems, vol. 35, pp. 24824–24837 (2022)

19. Zhou, D., et al.: Least-to-most prompting enables complex reasoning in large language models. arXiv preprint arXiv:2205.10625 (2022)
20. Zhang, Z., Zhang, A., Li, M., Smola, A.: Automatic chain of thought prompting in large language models. arXiv preprint arXiv:2210.03493 (2022)
21. Kojima, T., Gu, S.S., Reid, M., Matsuo, Y., Iwasawa, Y.: Large language models are zero-shot reasoners. In: Advances in Neural Information Processing Systems, vol. 35, pp. 22199–22213 (2022)
22. Zelikman, E., Wu, Y., Mu, J., Goodman, N.: STaR: bootstrapping reasoning with reasoning. In: Advances in Neural Information Processing Systems, vol. 35, pp. 15476–15488 (2022)
23. Hu, Z., et al.: LLM-adapters: an adapter family for parameter-efficient fine-tuning of large language models. arXiv preprint arXiv:2304.01933 (2023)
24. Li, X.L., Liang, P.: Prefix-tuning: optimizing continuous prompts for generation. arXiv preprint arXiv:2101.00190 (2021)
25. Dettmers, T., Pagnoni, A., Holtzman, A., Zettlemoyer, L.: QLORA: efficient fine-tuning of quantized LLMs. arXiv preprint arXiv:2305.14314 (2023)

Medical Knowledge Q&A Evaluation Based on ChatGPT Ensemble Learning

Pengbo Duan[✉] and Xin Su

School of Computer and Information Technology, Beijing Jiaotong University,
Beijing 100044, China
{pbduan,xinsue}@bjtu.edu.cn

Abstract. In the medical field, there is a large amount of clinical medical data, and a lot of knowledge is hidden in it. In recent years, the rapid development of Large Language Models (LLMs) has also affected the development of the medical field. And the application of LLMs has made computer-aided medical diagnosis possible. However, it is critical to ensure the accuracy and reliability of these models in clinical applications. This paper describes our participation in Task 4 of the China Conference on Health Information Processing (CHIP 2023). We propose a framework based on ChatGPT fusion ensemble learning to achieve question answering in medical domain. Experimental results show that our framework has excellent performance, with the Precision of 0.77, the Recall of 0.76, and the F1 of 0.76 in test dataset.

Keywords: Medical QA · Prompt Learning · Large Language Model · Ensemble Learning

1 Introduction

In the modern medical field, with the rapid development of AI technology, the application of medical Large Language Models (LLMs) has become an important tool for improving patient care and diagnosis. These models support doctors for more accurate diagnosis and treatment through advanced algorithms and large-scale data analysis. However, to ensure the maximum utility of these models in real-world clinical environments, their accuracy and reliability are indispensable.

The 9th China Health Information Processing Conference (CHIP2023) organized Evaluation Task 4, which aims to evaluate the performance of medical LLMs in dealing with complex medical problems. Through the evaluation of medical LLMs, the task is conducted to test their performance in medical fields such as medical terminology, medical knowledge, clinical standardized diagnosis and treatment, and medical computing. The main tasks cover the following aspects: the model needs to accurately understand and reasonably deduce medical terminology and knowledge; the model must be able to calculate and derive

---

P. Duan and X. Su—Contributed equally to this work.

H. Xu et al. (Eds.): CHIP 2023, CCIS 2080, pp. 148–155, 2024.
https://doi.org/10.1007/978-981-97-1717-0_13

based on medical formulas, accurately grasp patient symptoms, and provide appropriate professional clinical diagnosis and treatment knowledge.

Through these tasks, we are not only able to evaluate the preparation of medical LLMs in terms of theoretical knowledge, but also to consider their practicality and effectiveness in practical clinical applications. This evaluation is crucial for ensuring the safety and effectiveness of medical AI technology, and also provides valuable guidance and feedback for the future development of medical AI technology.

This paper focuses on evaluation task 4 and designs a framework based on ChatGPT fusion ensemble learning to complete knowledge Question Answering (QA). The framework mainly evaluates the ability of the GPT-4 model to solve medical knowledge QA. We design a series of prompt templates, ask questions for the ChatGPT and generate corresponding answers. We further regularize and integrally vote on the answers. Finally, we obtained an F1 score of 0.76 in the test dataset.

2   Related Work

2.1   Medical-Domain LLMs

With the rapid iteration of emerging technologies in LLMs, a series of LLMs such as GPT-3 [2], Instrument-GPT [12], and the recent birth of ChatGPT have demonstrated strong general-purpose language processing capabilities, achieving good performance with zero-shot or few-shot settings on various NLP tasks. At present, in the field of NLP, the paradigm of "Pre- train+Fine-tuning" is gradually being replaced by the paradigm of "Pre-train, Prompt, and Prediction". At present, many attempts have been made to fine-tune large models in specific domain like applying LLMs to the medical field. For example, DoctorGLM [19] and ChatDoctor [11] respectively monitor and fine-tune ChatGLM [3] and LLaMA [17] based on doctor-patient dialogue data. HuatuoGPT [21] uses over 160000 medical QA pairs for fine-tuning, which come from a diverse medical corpus. Clinicalcamel [16] combines doctor patient dialogue, clinical literature, and medical QA pairs to fine-tune the LLaMA2 model. Meanwhile, BenTsao [18] constructs knowledge-based instruction data from a knowledge graph. Zhongjing [20] further combines multiple rounds of dialogue as instruction data to perform fine-tuning.

2.2   Medical Question Answering

Automatic question answering (QA) has the ability to automatically answer a given question. In the field of biomedicine, QA systems can be used to assist in clinical decision support, create medical chat robots, and facilitate patient health. Over the past decade, a wide range of biomedical QA datasets have been introduced, including MedMCQA [13], MedQA (USMLE) [9], PubMedQA [10] and others. MedMCQA [13] and MedQA [9] are general medical knowledge tests in the United States Medical Licensing Examination (USMLE) and the Indian Medical Entrance Examination.

With the emergence of powerful LLMs, prompt based methods have been introduced to solve various QA tasks. For example, LLM Med-PaLM 2 [15] achieved a score of up to 86.5% on the USMLE dataset, surpassing Med-PaLM [14]. This LLM also exceeds the latest technological level in the clinical thematic datasets of MedMCQA [13], PubMedQA [10] and MMLU [8]. In the study [7], patient specific QA from clinical records were investigated using Chat-GPT, Google Bard, and Claude. The accuracy, relevance, comprehensiveness, and coherence of the answers generated by each model were evaluated using the 5-point Likert scale. Another study [6] proposes a retrieval based medical QA system that utilizes LLMs combined with knowledge graph to address challenge.

2.3 Ensemble Learning

Ensemble Learning is the process of combining the predicted results of models obtained from different algorithms in a certain way, taking the best of each model, in order to obtain model results that perform better than any single model.

The concept of ensemble learning can be traced back to Michael Kearns' paper in 1988. Leo Breiman [1] further developed this concept in his 1996 work by introducing "bagging" technology, known as bootstrap aggregation, to reduce the variance of individual models. Afterwards, Yoav Freund et al. [5] proposed another ensemble learning technique called "AdaBoost", which improves overall performance by focusing on instances where the previous model failed to classify correctly. In recent years, ensemble learning has been applied in multiple fields, including but not limited to bioinformatics, computer vision, and speech recognition. For example, Fernández Delgado et al. [4] compared 179 different classifiers, including multiple ensemble methods and found these ensemble learning methods typically outperform.

3   Methods

The overall framework of our study is shown in Fig. 1, including three distinct modules: the Prompt Design Module, the Regularization Processing Module and the Ensemble Learning Module.

Our approach begins with several prompt templates tailored to this evaluation task, with ChatGPT at the core. For each question-answering pair, these templates are employed to generate multiple results (n times). To ensure control over the model's outputs, we apply a regular expression processing, selectively retaining only the answers. In the final stage, we engage in an ensemble learning process, utilizing a majority vote strategy. This process involves collating the n answers generated for each question and electing the most representative answer as the final output.

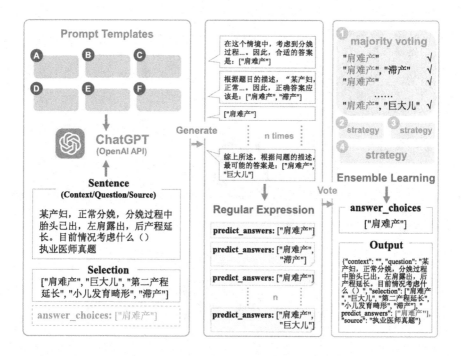

Fig. 1. The overview of our method.

3.1 Prompting

In the prompt template designing stage, we have designed several simple prompt templates, as shown in the Fig. 2. Firstly, We design the prompt templates for role-playing and define the system-role setting of ChatGPT as "You are a professional clinical expert." or "I hope you play an AI assisted doctor...". The remaining template is used to generate all multiple-choice prompts, and the elements in braces "{ }" will be replaced with specific values in the dataset.

3.2 Regular Expression Processing

Due to the fact that the answers generated by the large model may contain explanatory language, we use regular expressions to process the output results. Figure 3 shows an example question using a prompt template, where case 1 and case 2 are examples of model responses. We only extract the answers required in the prompt words within square brackets "[ ]", for example, in case 1, we extracted "肩难产" within square brackets; For cases that cannot match "[ ]" like Case2, we return an "Error" result.

{'''{question} ？ \n\n给定的答案选项列表：{selection}\n\n请从给定的答案列表中选出所有符合题目的答案选项，可能为多个。\n按照列表形式回复，如 ["答案1"，"答案2"，......]'''}

...

...

{'''这是一道{source}\n{question}？\n从下面的选项{selection}中选出所有符合题目的答案选项，请注意可能为多选。\n按照列表形式回复，如 ["答案1"，"答案2"，......] '''}

{'''题干问题：{question}？\n\n题干对应的候选文本项：{selection}\n请从中选出所有符合题目的答案选项，请注意可能为多选。\n按照列表形式回复，如 ["答案1"，"答案2"，......]'''}

You are a prefessional clinical expert.

我希望你扮演一个人工智能辅助医生。我将为您提供患者的详细信息，您的任务是使用最新的人工智能工具和医学领域知识，例如医学书籍和临床病例报告，对医学术语、医学知识、临床规范诊疗和医学计算进行理解和逻辑推理。准确把握患者症状，并提供恰如其分的专业临床诊疗知识.

Fig. 2. Template used to generate prompts.

Sample question using prompt template

{
题干问题："某产妇，正常分娩，分娩过程中胎头已出，左肩露出，后产程延长。目前情况考虑什么？"
题干对应的候选文本项：["肩难产"，"巨大儿"，"第二产程延长"，"小儿发育畸形"，"滞产"]
请从中选出所有符合题目的答案选项，请注意可能为多选。
按照列表形式回复，如 ["答案1"，"答案2"，……]
}

Case1：根据题干描述的情况：某产妇，正常分娩，分娩过程中胎头已出，左肩露出，后产程延长。我们可以考虑以下答案：
"肩难产"：当胎儿的头已通过母亲的骨盆，但是胎儿的肩部卡住而不能通过时，称为肩难产。所以，答案是：["肩难产"]。

Case2：根据题干描述，产妇经过正常分娩，胎头已出但随后产程延长，这种情况最有可能考虑的是"肩难产"。"小儿发育畸形"和"滞产"也可能导致产程延长，但根据题干中描述的具体情况，"肩难产"是最直接相关的选项。

Fig. 3. Sample question using prompt template.

3.3 Ensemble Voting

The predicted results of one single ChatGPT model have issues such as semantic inaccuracy and short-term memory of information. In order to further improve performance, this paper proposes an ensemble learning strategy, which adopts the simplest ensemble method of majority voting. This strategy integrates multiple ChatGPT generated result voting to improve accuracy.

4 Experiments

4.1 Dataset

The dataset utilized in this study is derived from the CHIP2023 Evaluation Task 4, which encompasses a broad spectrum of variables including a variety of diseases, the severity of these conditions and diverse patient demographics. This dataset comprises a series of multiple-choice questions meticulously curated from authentic clinical scenarios. These questions are sourced from an array of reputable resources: medical postgraduate entrance examination materials, queries typically encountered by practicing clinicians, authoritative medical textbooks, peer-reviewed medical literature and guidelines, as well as anonymized public medical records. The dataset is divided into two subsets: the training set, which contains 1,000 data, and 500 data in the testing set.

4.2 Evaluation Indicators

The experimental evaluation indicators include Precision, Recall, and F1 Score. Due to the multiple options in the dataset, this evaluation adopts the Micro Average F1 score as the evaluation indicator.

By adding up the number of true (TP), false positive (FP), and false negative (FN) examples of all answers, the overall Precision, recall, and F1 score are calculated as follows:

$$Precision = \frac{TP}{TP + FP} \tag{1}$$

$$Recall = \frac{TP}{TP + FN} \tag{2}$$

$$F1 = 2 \times \frac{Precision \times Recall}{Precision + Recall} \tag{3}$$

4.3 Results

Based on a single validation run using different models (HuatuoGPT, ChatGPT) on the labeled training dataset of 1000, the results are as shown in the Table 1. We observed that the performance with GPT-4 was superior. The precision reached 0.6117, recall reached 0.5888, and the F1 score was 0.6. Building on these findings, we utilized an ensemble-based ChatGPT as our evaluation model to call GPT-4's API on the test dataset. This approach reached the Precision of 0.77, the recall of 0.76, and the F1 score of 0.76.

Table 1. The results of different models on the dataset.

Dataset	Models	Precision	Recall	F1
Train	HuatuoGPT	0.3666	0.3022	0.3313
	GPT-4	0.6117	0.5888	0.6000
Test	GPT-4	0.7699	0.7594	0.7646

5 Conclusion

In recent years, Large Language Models (LLMs) have made significant strides in the field of Natural Language Processing, paving the way for their application in medicine. This paper proposed a framework based on ChatGPT fusion ensemble learning to achieve question answering in medical domain. This framework validated the feasibility of using LLMs prompt learning in medical knowledge question-answering scenarios, as well as the effectiveness of combining ensemble learning for voting on prediction results.

In the future, we will focus on fine-tuning large language models. We plan to explore the application of reinforcement learning and prompt learning in fine-tuning a large Chinese medical knowledge model.

References

1. Breiman, L.: Bagging predictors. Mach. Learn. **24**, 123–140 (1996)
2. Brown, T., et al.: Language models are few-shot learners. Adv. Neural. Inf. Process. Syst. **33**, 1877–1901 (2020)
3. Du, Z., et al.: GLM: general language model pretraining with autoregressive blank infilling. arXiv preprint arXiv:2103.10360 (2021)
4. Fernández-Delgado, M., Cernadas, E., Barro, S., Amorim, D.: Do we need hundreds of classifiers to solve real world classification problems? J. Mach. Learn. Res. **15**(1), 3133–3181 (2014)
5. Freund, Y., Schapire, R.E.: A decision-theoretic generalization of on-line learning and an application to boosting. J. Comput. Syst. Sci. **55**(1), 119–139 (1997)
6. Guo, Q., Cao, S., Yi, Z.: A medical question answering system using large language models and knowledge graphs. Int. J. Intell. Syst. **37**(11), 8548–8564 (2022)
7. Hamidi, A., Roberts, K.: Evaluation of AI chatbots for patient-specific EHR questions. arXiv preprint arXiv:2306.02549 (2023)
8. Hendrycks, D., et al.: Measuring massive multitask language understanding. arXiv preprint arXiv:2009.03300 (2020)
9. Jin, D., Pan, E., Oufattole, N., Weng, W.H., Fang, H., Szolovits, P.: What disease does this patient have? A large-scale open domain question answering dataset from medical exams. Appl. Sci. **11**(14), 6421 (2021)
10. Jin, Q., Dhingra, B., Liu, Z., Cohen, W.W., Lu, X.: PubMedQA: a dataset for biomedical research question answering. arXiv preprint arXiv:1909.06146 (2019)
11. Li, Y., Li, Z., Zhang, K., Dan, R., Jiang, S., Zhang, Y.: ChatDoctor: a medical chat model fine-tuned on a large language model meta-AI (LLaMA) using medical domain knowledge. Cureus **15**(6) (2023)

12. Ouyang, L., et al.: Training language models to follow instructions with human feedback. Adv. Neural. Inf. Process. Syst. **35**, 27730–27744 (2022)
13. Pal, A., Umapathi, L.K., Sankarasubbu, M.: MedMCQA: a large-scale multi-subject multi-choice dataset for medical domain question answering. In: Conference on Health, Inference, and Learning, pp. 248–260. PMLR (2022)
14. Singhal, K., et al.: Large language models encode clinical knowledge. arXiv preprint arXiv:2212.13138 (2022)
15. Singhal, K., et al.: Towards expert-level medical question answering with large language models. arXiv preprint arXiv:2305.09617 (2023)
16. Toma, A., Lawler, P.R., Ba, J., Krishnan, R.G., Rubin, B.B., Wang, B.: Clinical camel: an open-source expert-level medical language model with dialogue-based knowledge encoding. arXiv preprint arXiv:2305.12031 (2023)
17. Touvron, H., et al.: LLaMA: open and efficient foundation language models. arXiv preprint arXiv:2302.13971 (2023)
18. Wang, H., et al.: HuaTuo: tuning llama model with chinese medical knowledge. arXiv preprint arXiv:2304.06975 (2023)
19. Xiong, H., et al.: DoctorGLM: fine-tuning your Chinese doctor is not a herculean task. arXiv preprint arXiv:2304.01097 (2023)
20. Yang, S., et al.: Zhongjing: enhancing the chinese medical capabilities of large language model through expert feedback and real-world multi-turn dialogue. arXiv preprint arXiv:2308.03549 (2023)
21. Zhang, H., et al.: HuatuoGPT, towards taming language model to be a doctor. arXiv preprint arXiv:2305.15075 (2023)

Medical Literature PICOS Identification

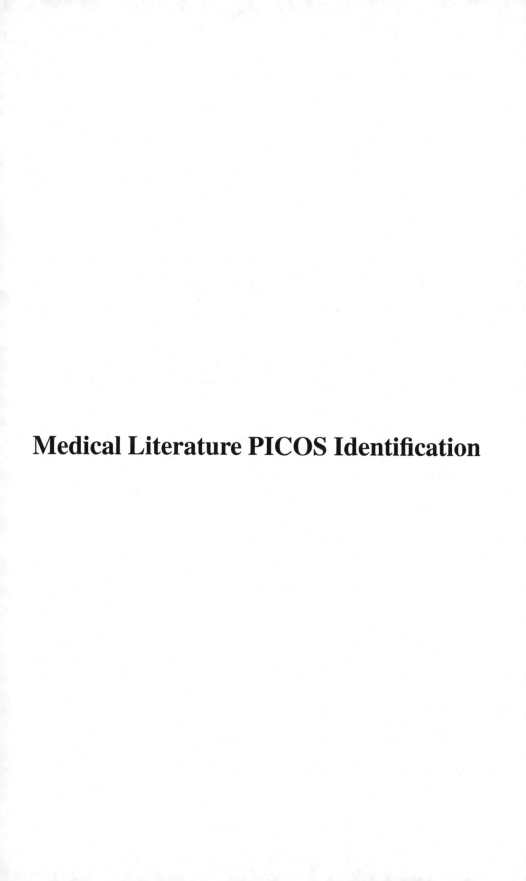

Overview of CHIP 2023 Shared Task 5: Medical Literature PICOS Identification

Hui Zong[1], Kangping Yin[2], Yixuan Tong[2], Zhenxin Ma[2], Jian Xu[2(✉)], and Buzhou Tang[3,4]

[1] West China Hospital, Sichuan University, Chengdu 610041, Sichuan, China
[2] Alibaba Group, Hangzhou 310000, Zhejiang, China
jian.xujian@alibaba-inc.com
[3] Harbin Institute of Technology (Shenzhen), Shenzhen 518055, Guangdong, China
[4] Pengcheng Laboratory, Shenzhen 518055, Guangdong, China

Abstract. Evidence-based medicine has become widely adopted among medical professionals, emphasizing the need for efficient information retrieval and evidence-based clinical practice. The PICOS framework, which stands for Population, Intervention, Comparison, Outcome, and Study design, has gained popularity as a structured approach for formulating research questions and retrieving relevant literature. In this paper, we present an overview of the "Medical Literature PICOS Identification" task organized at the CHIP 2023. The task aims to develop automated systems that accurately extract key information related to the PICOS components from Chinese medical research papers. The dataset consists of 4500 academic papers, divided into training, development, and test sets. Macro-F1 score are used as evaluation metric. Thirteen participating teams submitted their solutions, with the top-ranked team achieving a score of 0.81. This paper provides valuable insights into the challenges, methodologies, and performance of the top-ranked teams, serving as a resource for future research and system development in this domain.

Keywords: Information extraction · Large language model · PICOS · CHIP

1 Introduction

In recent years, evidence-based medicine has gained significant recognition and adoption among medical professionals as a guiding principle for learning and practice [1, 2]. With the advancement of medical informatics and databases, healthcare practitioners increasingly rely on evidence-based approaches to inform their decision-making processes. As a result, efficient information retrieval methods have become crucial in the field of evidence-based medicine. One such method that has gained considerable popularity is the PICOS framework, which stands for Population, Intervention, Comparison, Outcome, and Study design. The PICOS framework provides a structured approach to formulate research questions and retrieve relevant literature, thereby enhancing the efficiency and effectiveness of evidence-based searches.

H. Xu et al. (Eds.): CHIP 2023, CCIS 2080, pp. 159–165, 2024.
https://doi.org/10.1007/978-981-97-1717-0_14

Following the success of previous shared tasks at the Chine Health Information Processing Conference (CHIP) [3–5], such as the "Classifying Positive and Negative Clinical Findings in Medical Dialog" task in 2021 and the "Medical Causal Entity Relationship Extraction" task in 2022 [6], the Alibaba Quark Health Medical team introduce the "Medical Literature PICOS Identification" task at the CHIP 2023. The objective of this task is to develop automated systems that can accurately identify and extract key information related to the PICOS components from medical research articles. These components include the population under study, the specific intervention or treatment being investigated, the comparison group or alternative intervention, the desired clinical outcomes, and the study design employed in the research.

In this paper, we present an overview of the "Medical Literature PICOS Identification" task organized in CHIP 2023. Firstly, we provide an introduction to the task background and relevant studies, discussing the challenges involved in developing accurate and robust PICOS identification systems. Then, we describe the competition design, data collection, data annotation, dataset distribution, and evaluation metrics for this task. Finally, we present an overview of the overall participation and highlight the approaches employed by the top-ranked teams in the shared task.

2   Related Work

In 1995, the PICO framework was introduced [7], which offers a well-defined structure for conducting evidence-based research. To further enhance the application of the PICO framework, Kim et al. [8] constructed a manually annotated corpus comprising 1000 medical abstracts. This corpus was categorized into specific medical categories, including Background, Population, Intervention, Outcome, and Study Design. Nye et al. published the EBM-NLP corpus [9], which consisted of 5000 abstracts from medical articles describing clinical randomized controlled trials. The annotations in this corpus were more comprehensive, providing demarcations of text spans for the Patient population, Interventions, Comparisons, and Outcomes. This richly annotated corpus served as a valuable resource for training and evaluating information extraction models.

Several information extraction techniques have been investigated to identify the PICOS elements. In an earlier study [10], a classifier was developed using MetaMap [11], hand-written rules, and statistically derived features to extract the population, intervention, and outcome elements. In recent years, deep learning models have garnered considerable attention for their effectiveness in information extraction tasks. Researchers have successfully employed various techniques, including convolutional neural networks, bidirectional long short-term memory networks, and pretrained language models, to identify PICO elements. Furthermore, the evaluation of Easy Data Augmentation, a methodology that incorporates the vast knowledge of the Unified Medical Language System [12], has shown promise in PICO extraction. Recently, a study [13] released the EBM-NLP-mod dataset, which is derived from the EBM-NLP corpus. This dataset consists of 500 randomly selected abstracts from randomized controlled trials (RCTs), with re-annotated PICO elements. Additionally, two disease-specific datasets focused on Alzheimer's disease and COVID-19 were introduced, each containing 150 RCT abstracts annotated with PICO elements. To extract the PICO elements from RCT abstracts, the authors proposed a two-step NLP pipeline [13]. The first step involved sentence classification using a prompt-based learning model, while the second step utilized a named entity recognition model for PICO extraction.

3 Dataset

3.1 Task Definition

The data in this shared task is obtained from the titles and abstracts of Chinese academic literature. The objective of this task is to extract PICOS information, which stands for Population, Intervention, Comparison, Outcome, and Study design. In the realm of academic literature retrieval, most searches depend on keywords. Within this context, search keywords play two crucial roles. Firstly, they serve as indicators of the medical intention of the study, which involves a classification task. Secondly, they provide clinical information pertaining to the keywords associated with PICOS (Population, Intervention, Comparison, Outcome, Study design), thereby facilitating the identification of mentions in the title.

Here, we introduce the principle for the extraction of PICOS information. The "P" refers to the target population of the study, representing a specific group of individuals with a particular medical condition. The "I" denotes the intervention measures, representing the treatment plan or exposure factors for the intervention group. The "C" represents the comparison measures, which denote the treatment plan or exposure factors for the control group. The "O" signifies the outcome of interest, referring to important clinical outcomes such as effectiveness and survival rate. Finally, the "S" corresponds to the study design, indicating the types of study, whether it is a randomized controlled trial, cohort study, case-control study, or other types of studies.

3.2 Data Annotation

Based on upper considerations, we annotate the title and abstract separately. For the title, we first annotate study types, including treatment, diagnosis, etiology, prognosis, clinical statistics, and guideline recommendations. Second, we also annotate some key elements mentioned in title, such as the study population (P), intervention (I), outcome measures and assessment methods (O). For the abstract, the main purpose is to perform sentence-level text classification. Therefore, we annotate the categories, including study objectives, study methods, quantitative conclusion, and qualitative conclusion. Table 1 shows the detailed annotated labels, and Fig. 1 is an annotation example.

In this shared task, the dataset consists of a total of 4500 academic papers, including titles and abstracts. As shown in Table 2, the dataset is divided into three subsets: a training set of 2000 papers, a validation set of 500 papers, and a test set of 2000 papers. The test set is further divided into two parts: the leaderboard A and the leaderboard B. Each leaderboard contains 1000 papers. The leaderboard A is intended for participating teams to develop and optimize their algorithms during the competition, while the final competition ranking results are based on the leaderboard B. The dataset is stored in JSON format.

Table 1. The label types of population (P), intervention (I), comparison (C), outcome (O) and study design (S).

Types	Labels (Chinese)	Labels (English)
Population (P)	P-人群/患者类型 P-评估项 P-研究对象	P-Population/Patient Type P-Assessment Item P-Study Subject
Intervention (I)	I-药物干预 I-非药物干预 I-其他干预 I-教育/行为干预	I-Drug Intervention I-Non-Drug Intervention I-Other Intervention I-Education/Behavior Intervention
Comparison (C)	C-研究方法 C-研究目的	C-Study Method C-Study Objective
Outcome (O)	O-定性结论 O-定量结论	O-Qualitative Conclusion O-Quantitative Conclusion
Study design(S)	S-治疗 S-因素(病因/风险)分析 S-诊断 S-统计分析 S-预后	S-Treatment S-Factor (Etiology/Risk) Analysis S-Diagnosis S-Statistical Analysis S-Prognosis

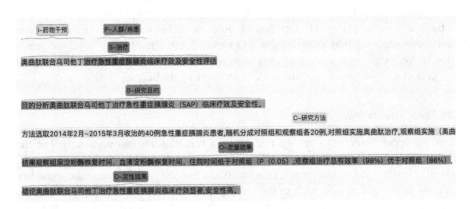

Fig. 1. Annotation example.

Table 2. Statistic of dataset for training, validation, and test.

Dataset	Training set	Validation set	Test set
Count	2000	500	2000

3.3 Evaluation Metrics

In this task, we use precision (P), recall (R), and F1 score as evaluation metrics. They are defined as follows: assuming there are n categories, Pi represents the precision of the i-th category, and Ri represents the recall of the i-th category.

$$\text{Macro} - \text{F1} = \frac{1}{n} \sum_{i=0}^{n} \frac{2 * P_i * R_i}{P_i + R_i}$$

In this task, Macro-F1 is used as the final evaluation metric. Considering the differences between title and abstract, a weighted approach is applied for ranking and the definition is as follows:

$$F1 = \frac{F1_{title} * 3 + F1_{abstract}}{4}$$

4 Results

4.1 Overview

The shared task is divided into two phases, namely the initial round (leaderboard A) and the final round (leaderboard B). The statistical results are presented in Table 3. A total of 13 submissions are received from participating teams for final ranking in leaderboard B. The highest achieved score is 0.81, while the lowest score recorded is 0.13. The average score among all teams is computed to be 0.69, with a median score of 0.77. Additionally, the standard deviation of scores is determined to be 0.20.

Table 3. Overall statistical result for all submission.

Phase	Submissions	Max	Min	Average	Median	Std
leaderboard A	19	0.7812	0.0753	0.5859	0.6179	0.1746
leaderboard B	13	0.8060	0.1270	0.6851	0.7727	0.1948

4.2 Top Three Solutions

Table 4 shows the results of the top three teams in this task. Here, we briefly introduce the algorithms used by the top three teams.

The first-ranked team proposed a Task-Specific Model Allocation approach for processing titles and abstracts data separately. Their model architecture consists of a title model and an abstract model. The title model uses a multi-task learning approach with an encoder layer, a span prediction layer using a Global Pointer Network (GPN) for entity recognition, and a classification layer to determine the category of the title. The abstract model primarily uses model fusion to enhance its robustness. In the abstracts

Table 4. The results of top three ranking teams.

Ranking	Score	Method
1st	0.8060	RoBERTa and Qwen
2nd	0.7978	Bert and ChatGLM
3th	0.7962	UIE and ERNIE-Health

model, the team combines models based on attention mechanisms (RoBERTa) and generative large-scale language models (Qwen) using a model fusion approach. They perform classification using the output of the CLS token from RoBERTa and apply supervised instruction fine-tuning using LORA on Qwen. A voting method is employed to combine the outputs of the models, and the model with the highest F1 score is chosen as the final result when the models produce inconsistent results.

The second ranked team proposes a framework for information extraction from medical text using BERT as the text classification module and ChatGLM as the entity extraction module. The framework includes task decomposition, where the "Abstract" text type is analyzed using text classification models, and the "Title" text type is treated as an entity recognition task. The information classification module utilizes RoBERT with adversarial training to improve classification accuracy for medical texts. The information extraction module employs ChatGLM with p-turning tuning to extract specific entities from medical texts. The framework aims to enhance the accuracy and robustness of information extraction from medical texts.

The third ranked team proposes a framework that integrates UIE (information extraction) and the ERNIE-Health model to extract critical information from medical literature. The UIE model is fine-tuned to extract elements of the PICOS principles, while the ERNIE-Health model is fine-tuned for precise classification. The team enhances the model's performance and robustness by introducing FGM and k-fold cross-validation. The approach focuses on information extraction precision, adaptability to medical contexts, and diverse data. The team also introduces a unified text-to-structure generation framework, UIE, to universally model different information extraction tasks. ERNIE-Health leverages medical domain understanding and has undergone extensive training with medical data. Fine-tuning is conducted on both models for key information extraction in medical papers.

5 Conclusion

This paper provides an overview of the "Medical Literature PICOS Identification" task organized by CHIP 2023. It includes the collection, annotation, and partitioning of the first dataset for extracting PICOS (Population, Intervention, Comparison, Outcome, Study design) information from Chinese medical literature, known as CHIP-PICOS. The paper also discusses the evaluation metrics, overall performance, and methodologies employed by the top-ranked teams in the task. In the future, researchers can further explore new algorithms on this dataset or develop systems for application in clinical practice.

References

1. Masic, I., Miokovic, M., Muhamedagic, B.: Evidence based medicine - new approaches and challenges. Acta Inform. Med. **16**(4), 219–225 (2008)
2. Djulbegovic, B., Guyatt, G.H.: Progress in evidence-based medicine: a quarter century on. Lancet **390**(10092), 415–423 (2017)
3. Zong, H., Lei, J., Li, Z.: Overview of technology evaluation dataset for medical multimodal information extraction. J. Med. Inform. **43**(12), 2–5 (2022)
4. Zhang, N., et al., CBLUE: a Chinese biomedical language understanding evaluation benchmark. ArXiv, abs/2106.08087 (2021)
5. Zong, H., et al.: Semantic categorization of Chinese eligibility criteria in clinical trials using machine learning methods. BMC Med. Inform. Decis. Mak. **21**(1), 128 (2021)
6. Li, Z., et al.: CHIP2022 shared task overview: medical causal entity relationship extraction. In: Tang, B., et al. (eds.) CHIP 2022. CCIS, vol. 1773, pp. 51–56. Springer, Singapore (2023). https://doi.org/10.1007/978-981-99-4826-0_5
7. Richardson, W.S., et al.: The well-built clinical question: a key to evidence-based decisions. ACP J. Club **123**(3), A12–A13 (1995)
8. Kim, S.N., et al., Automatic classification of sentences to support evidence based medicine. BMC Bioinform. **12 Suppl 2**(Suppl 2), S5 (2011)
9. Nye, B., et al.: A corpus with multi-level annotations of patients, interventions and outcomes to support language processing for medical literature. In: Proceedings of the Conference on Association for Computational Linguistics Meeting, vol. 2018, pp. 197–207 (2018)
10. Demner-Fushman, D., Lin, J.: Answering clinical questions with knowledge-based and statistical techniques. Comput. Linguist. **33**(1), 63–103 (2007)
11. Aronson, A.R., Lang, F.M.: An overview of MetaMap: historical perspective and recent advances. J. Am. Med. Inform. Assoc. **17**(3), 229–236 (2010)
12. Bodenreider, O.: The unified medical language system (UMLS): integrating biomedical terminology. Nucleic Acids Res. **32**(Database issue), D267–D270 (2004)
13. Hu, Y., et al.: Towards precise PICO extraction from abstracts of randomized controlled trials using a section-specific learning approach. Bioinformatics **39**(9) (2023)

Task-Specific Model Allocation Medical Papers PICOS Information Extraction

Qi Zhang[1], Jing Qu[1], Qingbo Zhao[1], and Fuzhong Xue[1,2(✉)]

[1] Healthcare Big Data Research Institute, School of Public Health,
Cheeloo College of Medicine, Shandong University, Jinan, China
`xuefzh@sdu.edu.cn`

[2] Department of Biostatistics, School of Public Health, Cheeloo College of Medicine,
Shandong University, Jinan, China

Abstract. In the field of medical research, extracting PICOS information which includes population, intervention, Comparison, outcomes, and study design from medical papers, plays a significant role in improving search efficiency and guiding clinical practice. Based on the PICOS key information extraction task released from the China Health Information Processing Conference (CHIP 2023), we proposed a method based on Task-Specific Model Allocation, which selects different models according to the characteristics of the abstract and title data. Additionally, incorporating techniques such as multi-task learning and model fusion. Our method achieved first place on the leaderboard with an F1 score of 0.78 on List A and 0.81 on List B.

Keywords: PICOS · Natural Language Processing · Multi-Task Learning

1 Introduction

As the number of medical papers increases rapidly, the difficulty of manually searching and reading these papers becomes more challenging. To enhance the efficiency of paper searches, the United States National Library of Medicine (NLM) has designed and released the Medical Subject Headings (MeSH) [1]. By manually matching the main keywords of published papers to the MeSH terms for retrieval, this method enhances the efficiency, accuracy, and comprehensiveness of searching. However, the process of extracting keywords and matching to the MeSH terms is labor-intensive and can not clearly identify the position of MeSH terms in the papers. The PICOS [2] (P: Population, I: Intervention, C: Comparison, O: Outcome, S: Study Design) framework was introduced to clarify key information and find its position in papers. Extracting PICOS information from medical papers can help researchers, doctors, and students to quickly and accurately find papers related to specific clinical questions, especially in conducting systematic reviews or evidence-based medical research. However, manually extracting PICOS information from medical papers is time-consuming and costly, hence the development of automated approaches for extracting PICOS information from medical papers is crucial.

There have been several datasets constructed for the PICOS information extraction, such as the EBM PICO [3] and PubMed PICO Element Detection Dataset [4]. These datasets and related extraction models have significantly advanced the process of automated PICOS information extraction. However, these datasets are primarily in English, and their annotation methods are limited, focusing solely on PICOS elements extraction or classification, without a single dataset encompassing both. To address these limitations, the Quark Medical Team launched the "Medical Paper PICOS Key Information Extraction Task" as part of the 9th China Health Information Processing Conference (CHIP 2023). This task focuses on the automatic extraction of PICOS information from titles and abstracts of papers, and the annotating features are diverse. Specifically, for titles, the task requires mention detection, while also classifying the entire title, for abstracts, it requires classifying the sentences within them. The evaluation task released 2140 manually labeled medical papers that include titles and abstracts as training data and 500 unlabeled medical literature papers test data.

For this task, we adopted a strategy based on Task-Specific Model Allocation, which involved designing specialized models for extracting relevant information from titles and abstracts separately. For the titles, we utilized a multi-task learning approach to simultaneously perform entity recognition and sentence classification. For the abstracts, we adopted a model fusion method, combining a BERT model with a larger generative model. Ultimately, we achieved an F1 score of 0.7516 for titles and 0.972 for abstracts, with a weighted F1 score of 0.807 on the test set.

The following sections of this paper will cover Data Description, Related Work, Methods, Experiments, and Conclusions.

2   Data Description

The dataset is composed of two parts: titles and abstracts of papers. For the titles, the task involves named entity recognition, with the entity categories being Population and Intervention. Additionally, the titles need to be classified, with title categories being Study Design, each of which has several subcategories. For the abstracts, the task is sentence-level classification, with sentence categories being Comparison and Outcome. Upon analyzing the data, we observed the following:

a) Different Tasks for Titles and Abstracts: tasks for titles involve named entity recognition and sentence-level classification, whereas task for abstracts involve only sentence-level classification.

b) Variations in Entity and Sentence Categories: The entity categories and sentence categories for titles and sentence categories for abstracts differ significantly, making it impractical to use the same labels for definition

c) Significant Length Differences: The maximum length of titles is 54 characters with an average length of 23.7 characters. In contrast, The maximum length of abstracts is 1180 characters, with an average length of 364.8 characters.

d) Inconsistencies in Annotation: For instance, in the title "女性狼疮患者生活质量与家庭婚姻功能的相关性研究", "女性狼疮患者" is labeled as "P-Population/Patient Type". However, in "血管内皮生长因子表达水平与宫颈癌患者预后的关系", only "宫颈癌" is labeled as "P-Population/Patient Type", omitting the word "患者". Additionally, there are a few annotation errors.

As the data features mentioned above, although the titles and abstracts in the dataset correspond to each other, allowing for the identification of the abstract for each title and thus providing complementary information to some extent. Considering the significant differences in task types, categories, and text lengths between these two parts, we decided not to use a single model or data fusion approach for model design. Instead, we chose to design distinct models for titles and abstracts, allowing for more targeted training and optimization.

3 Related Work

There has been much research on the automatic extraction methods of PICO. Earlier researches primarily based on rule-based methods. For example, Demner-Fushman et al. [5] proposed a method based on specified rules, using UMLS and MetaMap to identify PICO elements. However, these methods were time-consuming, labor-intensive, and had limited generalizability. Subsequently, many machine learning algorithms, such as Support Vector Machines [6] and Conditional Random Fields [7], were also used for PICO information extraction, but these methods often required the addition of specific rules. With the advent of deep learning, which showed advantages in natural language processing like eliminating the need for manually crafted features and capturing deep semantic information, researchers have increasingly turned to deep learning models for automatic PICO extraction. Jin et al. [4] treated PICO information detection as a sequential sentence classification task, using Bi-directional Long Short-Term Memory (bi-LSTM) to gather contextual information from sentences, thereby improving predictions for the current sentence. Zhang T et al. [8] employed various frameworks such as BERT and CNN, adopting a step-wise approach for sentence classification and extraction of P and I type entities. Hu Y et al. [9] also used a two-step approach for PICO extraction, combining classification and named entity recognition, and introduced prompt learning. Dhrangadhariya A et al. [10] proposed a 'DISTANT-CTO' method aimed at improving PICO entity extraction in low-resource settings, which involves generating a large dataset of weakly labeled data through distant supervision, thereby enhancing the extraction effectiveness of PICO.

Named Entity Recognition (NER) primarily employs sequence labeling methods and span-based methods. The sequence labeling approach identifies entities using schemes like BIO or BIOES, obtaining entity representations through models like BERT, and then deriving entity category probabilities through a linear layer or a CRF layer. While this method is relatively simple, it requires correctly predicting the category of each token, resulting in less effective predictions for longer entities and difficulties in addressing nested and discontinuous entities. The span-based methods for obtaining entities by assessing entity boundaries primarily include the following approaches: enumerating all possible spans within a sentence to determine mentions, generating labels using pointer networks, and employing the Machine Reading Comprehension (MRC) approach. Based on the pointer network approach, which offers greater flexibility, many of the currently more effective models employ this method for named entity recognition. For instance, the Biaffine model, which effectively addresses nested entities by constructing a head-tail entity matrix and obtaining the score for each span through a biaffine mechanism, Yu J et al. [11] utilized this to establish syntactic relationships. Global Pointer [12] introduces a global pointer network, computing the score of each span through multiplicative attention. Additionally, it incorporates relative position encoding. This model has been widely applied in various NER competitions. Additionally, W2NER [13] effectively addresses the issue of discontinuous entities by introducing two types of relationships between words: NNW and THW. This approach has achieved state-of-the-art results in various tasks.

The mainstream approach to text classification involves using an encoder to obtain a sentence representation, followed by adding a Classification Head that transforms the extracted sentence representation into class probabilities. Encoders can be models based on CNN (e.g., TextCNN [14]), RNN, GCN, and attention mechanism-based models like BERT. In the case of BERT, sentence representations are typically obtained through the CLS layer, average pooling, or max pooling. In recent years, methods like Weighted Pooling, Attention Pooling, and the combination of multi-layer hidden states have also been used to extract sentence representations. The classification head often comprises a fully connected layer and a softmax layer. Recently, sentence classification methods involving contrastive learning, meta-learning [15], and reinforcement learning [16] have also been introduced. These novel approaches provide the potential for deeper analysis and classification of complex textual data, bringing new research directions and breakthroughs to the field of text classification.

Multi-task learning involves learning multiple related tasks simultaneously during the training phase. It is based on a core assumption: different tasks can share information, thereby enhancing the model's learning efficiency and generalization ability for each individual task. Typically, the model consists of a shared layer, where multiple tasks share a portion of the parameters, along with task-specific model layers unique to each task. Multi-task learning has been applied in various deep learning applications. For instance, Zhao R et al. [17] proposed a multi-task learning framework (MCL-Net) for multiple indices of the visual nerve. This framework first obtains task-shared and task-specific representations through a backbone network and two branch networks, followed by an interactive module that fuses the representations from both branches. Liu P et al. [18] introduced a framework for adversarial multi-task learning. Gan C et al. [19] utilized multi-task learning for simultaneous named entity recognition and sentence classification, employing a unified input format and a generative model to generate SC-labels, NER-labels, and associated text segments.

4   Method

Considering the differences between two types of data, we proposed the Task-Specific Model Allocation approach, using two separate models to process titles data and abstracts data. Our model architecture, as shown in Fig. 1, consists of a title model on the left, employing a multi-task learning approach made up of an encoder layer, a span prediction layer, and a classification layer. The

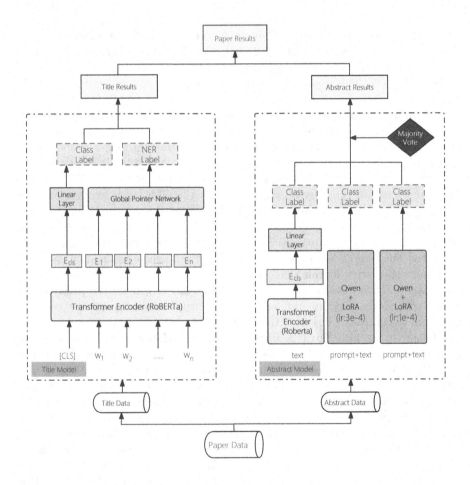

Fig. 1. Architecture of the model.

encoder layer uses the RoBERTa model [20] to obtain representations of tokens in the text; the span prediction layer employs a Global Pointer Network (GPN) for entity recognition, described in Sect. 4.1. The classification layer is used to determine the category of the title, detailed in Sect. 4.2. On the right side of Fig. 1 is the abstract model, which primarily uses model fusion to enhance the robustness of the model, detailed in Sect. 4.3.

4.1 Global Pointer Network

We adopted the global pointer network approach for entity extraction and classification, with the framework being Global Pointer(GP) [12], which was proposed by Su J et al., aiming to resolve issues encountered in traditional entity recognition methods when dealing with nested and long-span entities. The model primarily consists of a Token Representation layer and a Span Prediction layer. After obtaining sentence representation H, span representations are calculated. To this end, two feedforward layers are used, which operate based on the start and end indices of the span. Specifically, for each entity type α, two transformations $Wq\alpha$ and $Wk\alpha$ are employed to calculate the representations $qi\alpha$ and $ki\alpha$ for each token:

$$q_{i,\alpha} = W_{q,\alpha}h_i + b_{q,\alpha} \tag{1}$$

$$k_{i,\alpha} = W_{k,\alpha}h_i + b_{k,\alpha} \tag{2}$$

Then, the score for the span s[i:j] being an entity of type α is calculated, which is represented as:

$$s_\alpha(i,j) = q_{i,\alpha}^\top k_{j,\alpha} \tag{3}$$

Additionally, to leverage boundary information, the model explicitly incorporates relative position information into its framework. By applying the Rotary Positional Encoding (ROPE) to the entity representations, the resulting score function becomes:

$$s_\alpha(i,j) = \left(\mathcal{R}_i q_{i,\alpha}\right)^\top \left(\mathcal{R}_j k_{j,\alpha}\right) \tag{4}$$

where Ri and Rj are encodings based on the relative positions.

4.2 Classification Head

We used the output of the CLS token from the final layer of the encoder to predict the category of the sentence. For sentence category prediction, other methods like taking the logits output followed by average pooling or max pooling can also be employed. However, considering that the logits output requires further processing through a decoder for predicting token boundaries, using this data for sentence category prediction might affect the accuracy of boundary recognition.

Therefore, we opt to use only the CLS layer for sentence category prediction. The specific method involves passing the output of the CLS layer through a dropout layer, followed by a linear layer for classification.

In the model, the parameters of the encoder are shared between the span prediction task and the classification task, while the span prediction layer and the classification layer each adapt to their respective tasks. We use cross-entropy as the loss function for the classification. The total loss is calculated using a weighted sum approach. Considering that the classification task is relatively simple, The total loss is expressed as:

$$F1 = (\text{NER\_Loss} \times 2 + \text{SC\_Loss})/3 \tag{5}$$

4.3   Fusion Model

As for abstracts, we adopts a model fusion approach, comprising models based on attention mechanisms (RoBERTa) and generative large-scale language models (Qwen [21]), to evaluate their performance in classification tasks. For the RoBERTa model, used the output of the CLS token from the final layer of the encoder and classification is performed using an additional linear layer. On the QWEN model, supervised instruction fine-tuning is carried out using LORA [22]. The prompt is designed as: '请判断下面的医学语句属于哪个类别,可选的类别为:S-诊断,S-治疗,S-因素(病因/风险)分析,S-统计分析,S-预后。需要判断的句子是:XXX', where 'XXX' represents the sentence that needs classification. Finally, a voting method is employed, combining the outputs of RoBERTa, Qwen(lr:1e−4), and Qwen(lr:3e−4). When the three models produce inconsistent results, the output of the model with the highest F1 score is chosen as the final result.

5   Experiments

5.1   Data Preprocessing

We splited the labeled data into training data and evaluation data in a 9:1 ratio. The training data is used for model training, and the evaluation data is for assessing the model's effectiveness. Further, the data is divided into two datasets based on text type: a title dataset and an abstract dataset.

5.2   Evaluation Metrics

Using the Macro-F1 score as the evaluation metric, the formula is:

$$\text{Macro} - F1 = \frac{1}{n} \sum_{i=1}^{n} \frac{2 \times P_i \times R_i}{P_i + R_i} \tag{6}$$

where P represents precision, and R represents recall.

For the results of the title and abstract, the overall F1 score is calculated using a weighted F1 method, which is:

$$F1 = (\text{F1\_Title} \times 3 + \text{F1\_Abstract})/4 \tag{7}$$

5.3   Parameter Settings

In both the model used for titles and the RoBERTa model used for abstracts, we use the 'chinese-roberta-wwm-ext-large' model and select Adam as the optimizer, with a learning rate of 2e−5. The checkpoint with the highest F1 score on the evaluation data is saved. For the Qwen model for abstracts, we use Qwen-7b, which undergoes LoRA fine-tuning at two distinct learning rates: 1e−4 and 3e−4, over a training duration of 3 epochs.

5.4   Training Techniques

a) To enhance the model's performance, we incorporated adversarial training into both models. Adversarial training is a common technique that introduces noise to regularize model parameters, thereby enhancing the model's robustness and generalization capability. Specifically, we adopted the Fast Gradient Method (FGM) [23].

b) We utilized an iterative training approach to correct the question data in the training dataset. Specifically, we used pseudo-label data from the test set to train an additional model to make predictions on the training dataset. We then compared the discrepancies between the predicted and actual annotations, and manually corrected the inconsistent parts. The principle of modification was to address definite errors rather than ambiguous ones. For example, for the sentence "痰热清注射液治疗病毒性乙型肝炎疗效观察", the entity "痰热清" was added as "I-Medical Intervention", and the label of "胰腺癌组织" was changed from "P-Population/Patient Type" to "P-Study Subject".

5.5   Results

We conducted ablation study to demonstrate the effective of multi-task learning. The model's performance was evaluated in scenarios where only the NER module or the classification module was included. These evaluations were conducted on the evaluation dataset. The results showed that when performing individual tasks separately, the F1 score for the classification task was higher than that in multi-task learning, but the F1 score for the NER task was lower than the classification F1 score in multi-task learning. The overall F1 score in multi-task learning was higher than that of models performing each task separately. This indicates that multi-task learning can enhance the extraction effectiveness of PICOS elements. We observed that the multi-task model had relatively lower performance in the classification task, possibly because the classification task is simpler and can achieve good results with a single model. In contrast, Named Entity Recognition is more challenging, and multi-task learning, by fitting both the classification information and NER simultaneously, can aid in improving the extraction performance of NER.   The specific results are shown in Table 1. Simultaneously, we calculated the proportion of different mention categories under different sentence types in the title data and presented it in the form of a heatmap to observe whether there is a correlation between the two sets of data. The results, as shown in Fig. 2, indicate that there is a certain degree of correlation between the two types of data. Therefore, the information from one task can contribute to enhancing the prediction performance of another task.

Table 1. F1 scores with and without multitask learning.

Model	EPOCH	NER F1	SC F1	Overall F1
MTL	6	0.7882	0.912	0.8279
NER	4	0.7774	–	–
SC	4	–	0.9213	–
NER+SC	–	–	–	0.8197

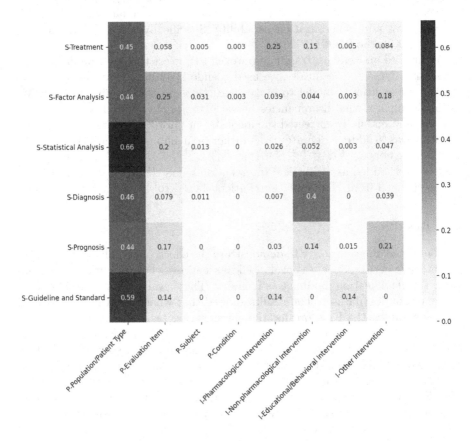

Fig. 2. Percentage of different mentions under different categories of the topic.

In the test dataset, we validated the title model and the abstract model separately and validated the overall performance of the model in the end. In the title model, different optimization methods all led to improvements in model performance. In the abstract model, the performance of the large language model was superior to that of the RoBERTa model. When the three were combined in a model fusion, the performance was optimal. The specific results are shown in Table 2:

Table 2. F1 scores under different technical methods.

Task	Technical Method	F1-score
Title	MTL+FGM+ Data Correction	0.7516
	MTL +FGM	0.7303
	MTL	0.7045
Abstract	Fusion Model	0.9724
	Qwen(1e−4)	0.9716
	Qwen(3e−4)	0.9708
	RoBERTa	0.9688
Overall	–	0.8068

6 Discussion

In this paper, we proposed a Task-Specific Model Allocation method tailored to extract PICOS information from medical papers. Specifically, we adopted a multi-task learning approach to address sentence classification and PICOS elements extraction in title tasks and employed optimization methods such as adversarial learning. For the classification of abstract sentences, we primarily used a model fusion approach. Our method achieved the first rank, demonstrating its effectiveness. Due to time constraints, we did not explore further possibilities. In the future, we plan to optimize the model further. For instance, since the F1 score for classification tasks without multi-task learning was higher than that with multi-task learning, we could use a two-phase model, first classifying and then extracting mentions, and experimenting with different pre-trained models, to further improve the model's performance.

References

1. Sayers, E.W., et al.: Database resources of the national center for biotechnology information. Nucleic Acids Res. **49**(D1), D10 (2021)
2. Richardson, W.S., Wilson, M.C., Nishikawa, J., Hayward, R.S.: The well-built clinical question: a key to evidence-based decisions. ACP J. Club **123**(3), A12–A13 (1995)

3. Nye, B., et al.: A corpus with multi-level annotations of patients, interventions and outcomes to support language processing for medical literature. In: Proceedings of the conference. Association for Computational Linguistics. Meeting, vol. 2018, p. 197. NIH Public Access (2018)

4. Jin, D., Szolovits, P.: Pico element detection in medical text via long short-term memory neural networks. In: Proceedings of the BioNLP 2018 Workshop, pp. 67–75 (2018)

5. Demner-Fushman, D., Lin, J.: Answering clinical questions with knowledge-based and statistical techniques. Comput. Linguist. **33**(1), 63–103 (2007)

6. McKnight, L., Srinivasan, P.: Categorization of sentence types in medical abstracts. In: AMIA Annual Symposium Proceedings, vol. 2003, p. 440. American Medical Informatics Association (2003)

7. Kim, S.N., Martinez, D., Cavedon, L., Yencken, L.: Automatic classification of sentences to support evidence based medicine. In: BMC Bioinformatics, vol. 12, pp. 1–10. BioMed Central (2011)

8. Zhang, T., Yu, Y., Mei, J., Tang, Z., Zhang, X., Li, S.: Unlocking the power of deep PICO extraction: step-wise medical NER identification. arXiv preprint arXiv:2005.06601 (2020)

9. Hu, Y., Keloth, V.K., Raja, K., Chen, Y., Xu, H.: Towards precise PICO extraction from abstracts of randomized controlled trials using a section-specific learning approach. Bioinformatics **39**(9), btad542 (2023)

10. Dhrangadhariya, A., Müller, H.: Distant-CTO: a zero cost, distantly supervised approach to improve low-resource entity extraction using clinical trials literature. In: Proceedings of the 21st Workshop on Biomedical Language Processing. Association for Computational Linguistics (2022)

11. Yu, J., Bohnet, B., Poesio, M.: Named entity recognition as dependency parsing. arXiv preprint arXiv:2005.07150 (2020)

12. Su, J., et al.: Global pointer: novel efficient span-based approach for named entity recognition. arXiv preprint arXiv:2208.03054 (2022)

13. Li, J., et al.: Unified named entity recognition as word-word relation classification. In: Proceedings of the AAAI Conference on Artificial Intelligence, vol. 36, pp. 10965–10973 (2022)

14. Gong, L., Ji, R.: What does a TextCNN learn? arXiv preprint arXiv:1801.06287 (2018)

15. Bao, Y., Wu, M., Chang, S., Barzilay, R.: Few-shot text classification with distributional signatures. arXiv preprint arXiv:1908.06039 (2019)

16. Zhang, T., Huang, M., Zhao, L.: Learning structured representation for text classification via reinforcement learning. In: Proceedings of the AAAI Conference on Artificial Intelligence, vol. 32 (2018)

17. Zhao, R., Li, S.: Multi-indices quantification of optic nerve head in fundus image via multitask collaborative learning. Med. Image Anal. **60**, 101593 (2020)

18. Liu, P., Qiu, X., Huang, X.: Adversarial multi-task learning for text classification. arXiv preprint arXiv:1704.05742 (2017)

19. Gan, C., Zhang, Q., Mori, T.: Sentence-to-label generation framework for multi-task learning of Japanese sentence classification and named entity recognition. In: Métais, E., Meziane, F., Sugumaran, V., Manning, W., Reiff-Marganiec, S. (eds.) NLDB 2023. LNCS, vol. 13913, pp. 257–270. Springer, Cham (2023). https://doi.org/10.1007/978-3-031-35320-8_18

20. Liu, Y., et al.: RoBERTa: a robustly optimized BERT pretraining approach. arXiv preprint arXiv:1907.11692 (2019)

21. Bai, J., et al.: Qwen technical report. arXiv preprint arXiv:2309.16609 (2023)
22. Hu, E.J., et al.: LoRA: low-rank adaptation of large language models. arXiv preprint arXiv:2106.09685 (2021)
23. Miyato, T., Dai, A.M., Goodfellow, I.: Adversarial training methods for semi-supervised text classification. arXiv preprint arXiv:1605.07725 (2016)

LLM Collaboration PLM Improves Critical Information Extraction Tasks in Medical Articles

Mengyuan Cao[1], Hang Wang[1], Xiaoming Liu[2(✉)], Jiahao Wu[3],
and Mengting Zhao[1,2,3]

[1] Zhongyuan University of Technology, Zhengzhou 450007, China
[2] Henan Key Laboratory on Public Opinion Intelligent Analysis, Zhengzhou 450007, China
ming616@zut.edu.cn
[3] Zhengzhou Key Laboratory of Text Processing and Image Understanding, Zhengzhou 450007, China

Abstract. With the development of modern medical informatics and databases, medical professionals are increasingly inclined to use evidence-based medicine to guide their learning and work. Evidence-based medicine requires a large amount of data and literature information, where most search processes are keyword retrieval. Therefore, anticipating these key information through the model can play an important role in optimizing the query. In the past, the PLM (Pre-trained Language Model) model was mainly used for information extraction, but due to the complexity of the sequence semantic structure and task diversity, it is difficult for traditional PLM to achieve the desired effect. With the advancement of LLM (Large Language Model) technology, these issues can now be well managed. In this paper, we discuss the information extraction evaluation task CHIP-PICOS, and finally decompose it into classification and information extraction sub-problems, applying PLM and LLM respectively, and analyzing the advantages and disadvantages and differences between PLM and LLM. The results show that our framework has achieved significant performance.

Keywords: Information extraction · PLM · Collaboration · LLM

1 Introduction

With the rapid development of medical informatics and databases, medical practitioners are facing the challenge of information explosion [1]. In the vast amount of information, it is crucial to quickly and accurately find the key information needed. This not only requires efficient query methods, but also needs to extract accurate and comprehensive key information from the database. In the past, it was mainly dealt with using methods based on general pre-training models. However, the effect of this method is not ideal. On the one hand, some annotated corpora are missing, the generalizability is not enough, semantics are relatively complex, and the extraction fields are too long, which greatly reduces the accuracy and efficiency of searching. On the other hand, this method cannot handle large-scale semantic information well, the system complexity is too large, which often results in a lack of comprehensiveness in the search results [2].

H. Xu et al. (Eds.): CHIP 2023, CCIS 2080, pp. 178–185, 2024.
https://doi.org/10.1007/978-981-97-1717-0_16

In recent years, in 2017, Google proposed the Transformer [3], which subverted the previous neural network structure and used attention mechanisms to improve model training speed and semantic understanding ability. Since then, large-scale pre-training language [4] models have also entered people's horizons due to their good performance in tasks such as machine translation, Q&A, information extraction, etc. With the vigorous development of deep learning and natural language processing technology, large models have achieved significant results in many fields. These large models, such as GPT-4, have stronger semantic understanding and reasoning capabilities, and can better handle complex semantic information and extract comprehensive key information. Therefore, applying large models to the query of medical informatics and databases can greatly improve the accuracy and efficiency of the query [5].

In addition, with the development of artificial intelligence technology, in the evolution process of big models, researchers have found that the performance of the models will increase correspondingly with the continuous increase of training data and parameters. The model parameter level has also jumped from the earliest billion level to the billion, trillion, and even the trillion model level. What follows is a leap in the model's universal capabilities. When the model parameters exceed a certain threshold, the model will "emerge" amazing understanding, reasoning, learning, etc. [6]. Therefore, when big models are applied to modern medical information extraction tasks, we can hope to achieve more intelligent medical information queries. For example, by using natural language generation technology, we can automatically organize the extracted key information into complete case reports, literature abstracts, etc.; by using natural language dialogue technology, we can realize smart questions and answers, intelligent guidance, etc., making medical information queries more convenient and efficient [7].

Therefore, the discriminative model represented by BERT [8] can no longer fully meet business needs. By applying large models, generative models have become a major trend in artificial intelligence technology. We can achieve more accurate and comprehensive key information queries, thereby providing better work support for medical practitioners and stronger data support for medical research and decision-making. At the same time, with the development of artificial intelligence technology, we can expect to achieve more intelligent and convenient medical information queries, making a greater contribution to the improvement of medical service quality [9].

2   Related Work

2.1   Information Extraction Method Based on Traditional Pre-training Models

The Information extraction methods based on traditional pre-training models are mainly done by classifying the key information to be extracted. For various sequence labeling tasks, fine-tuning is done on the pre-trained language model based on labeled training data. This method can effectively extract textual context semantic features, but its effect in recognizing various types of information may be limited in scenarios with complex information categories [16]. Fu et al. [10] take into account the interaction between entities and relations through relation-weighted GCN, but this cannot capture the global dependency relationships between tasks. REN [11] and others convert entity relation joint extraction into a table filling problem, establishing global associations versus the traditional focus on local associations. Parameter sharing methods set the underlayer or the middle layer parameters of the model as shared parameters to capture the shared features and patterns among multiple tasks. Miwa et al. [12] built an entity's sequence labeling model and relationship's dependency tree model respectively on the shared LSTM layer, establishing simple interaction between tasks through common encoding layer. Yan et al. [13] used partition filtration network to separate task-specific features and shared features between tasks, alleviating the feature conflict problem existing in the feature interaction process. Xu et al. [14] defined event relationship triplets through the event triggering words, arguments, and argument roles to learn their interdependencies. Feng et al. [15] designed a soft parameter sharing method for the event recognition task and argument role classification task based on the MMOE framework, controlling the information sharing between tasks at a more granular level using a gating mechanism.

The above research shows that joint extraction of information extraction sub-tasks leverages the synergy between tasks to further optimize the feature representation of sub-tasks, thus leading to overall performance improvement. However, current research on joint extraction is in line with the views of Zhong et al. [17]: pipeline models still show considerable performance in certain scenarios compared to joint models, and more exploration is needed for effective task cooperation mechanisms. In addition, current methods mostly focus on capturing the dependency relationship between tasks, neglecting the problem of knowledge negative transfer and imbalance between task feature specificity and sharedness in task interaction [18].

2.2 Information Extraction Methods Based on Large Models

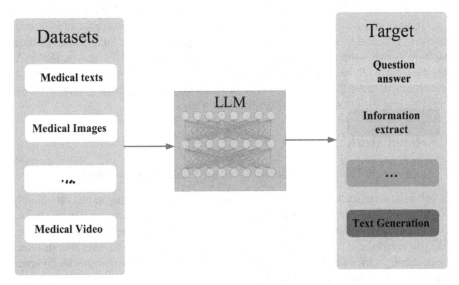

Fig. 1. Harmonisation of tasks downstream of the big model

As shown in Fig. 1, it is the base task architecture of large models, their outstanding general learning ability has given birth to a new paradigm of multi-task learning. The Universal Information Extraction Framework (UIE) proposed by Lu et al. [19] learns collaboratively from different knowledge sources, and unifies the different structures of multiple information tasks. Wei et al. [20] based on ChatGPT, proposed ChatIE to solve zero-shot information extraction tasks through multi-round question and answer dialogues, and explored the difficulty of extracting structured text with multiple dependencies in one-time predictions. These methods unify multiple information extraction tasks as text-to-structure generation tasks through a single framework, in order to capture the basic knowledge that can be shared among different extraction tasks, and have shown clear advantages in zero-shot and small-sample scenarios.

However, compared with fine-tuned models, they still fall short on many tasks and datasets under full supervision. Also, it is still unclear if the methods based on large models still suffer from the negative transfer problem commonly seen in multi-task learning, and how to deal with this problem needs further study. This may require further analysis and explanation of the interaction between multi-tasks relationships.

3   Proposed Framework

Throughout the entire research process, in order to make full use of the structural information in medical texts, this paper utilizes BERT as the text classification module, and ChatGLM as the entity extraction module. Figure 2 is a demonstration of the unified model process.

3.1   Task Decomposition

In the CHIP-ICOS dataset, there are two different types of text: one is "Abstract", which is a continuous piece of information requiring information extraction tasks, for which we choose to use a text classification model; the other is "Title", where the text needs to extract entity information from a sentence, so we consider this task as an application scenario for the entity recognition model. For the "Abstract" text type, the task we face is to extract key information from a sentence, this approach systematically categorizes and extracts key information from the continuous content present in the "Abstract" text type. We can use text classification models, such as deep learning-based models (such as BERT, LSTM, etc.), to analyze and extract "Abstract". For the "Title" text type, our goal is to extract entities from the title of a sentence.

This is a task of entity recognition, the model needs to be able to recognize specific entities in the text, which may involve Named Entity Recognition (NER) techniques. By adopting large model structures and training data, we can train a model that can accurately extract entities. This method of distinguishing tasks helps us choose the appropriate model and technology to more effectively solve different types of information extraction problems. At the same time, a reasonable task description also provides a clear goal for model training and evaluation, helping to ensure that the model can achieve the expected results in actual applications.

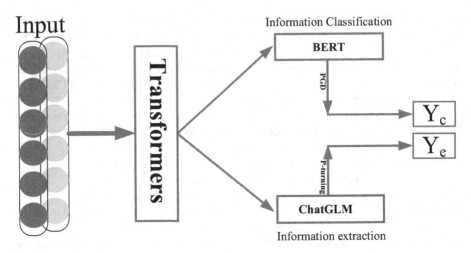

Fig. 2. Unified Healthcare Model Architecture

3.2 Information Classification Module

Given that information in medical texts often exists in continuous paragraphs, we choose to use a text classification model for information extraction. In the classification model of this paper, we use RoBERT as the base architecture, combined with Projected Gradient Descent (PGD) [21] for adversarial training, to improve the model's classification accuracy for medical texts. RoBERT [22], or Bidirectional Encoder Representations from Transformers for Robust Classification, is a strong pre-trained language model that captures context and semantic relationships in the text, providing strong support for the medical text classification task. By using PGD for adversarial training, we introduce adversarial perturbations to make the model more robust when facing disturbances in the input text. The Projected Gradient Descent optimization method of PGD helps generate adversarial samples, thus training the model to better adapt to the diversity and complexity of medical texts. The specific formula is as follows:

$$H_c = PGD(RoBert(X))$$
$$Y_c = Linner(W_c \cdot H_c + b_c)[0] \tag{1}$$

Among $X_1 = [x_1, x_2, \ldots, x_n]$, $H_c \in R^{n*d}$, $W_c \in R^{d*n}$, $b_p \in R^n$ and $Y_c \in R^c$, where n represents the number of tokens in the text, and c represents the number of classification labels. By combining RoBert with PGD, we hope to improve the model's performance in handling medical text classification tasks, making it more robust and generalizable. This method not only helps to accurately extract medical information, but also effectively deals with the noise and variants in the text, improving the reliability of the model in practical applications.

3.3 Information Extraction Module

In order to capture information in medical texts more finely, we chose ChatGLM [23] as our entity extraction tool. ChatGLM, as a powerful language generation model, is flexible and can handle the details of medical texts more delicately. We focus on the task of entity extraction, aiming to accurately and comprehensively extract specific entities from medical texts, such as diseases, drugs, etc., to meet more specific information needs. On this basis, we used p-turning tuning method, and ChatGLM was deeply optimized to focus on the task of entity extraction. This tuning method is carefully designed to adapt to the complex and diverse entity structures in the medical field. Our goal is to make the model more sensitive to various entities involved in medical texts, thereby improving the accuracy and breadth of information extraction. The specific calculations are as follows:

$$Y_e = Pturning(ChatGLM(X_2))) \tag{2}$$

where $X_2 = [x_1, x_2, \ldots, x_n]$ and, $Y_e \in R^{n*e}$ and e represents the type of entity. In general, we have built a large-scale model focused on the task of entity extraction, combining the language generation capabilities of ChatGLM and the optimization strategy of p-turning tuning [24]. This model aims to realize more meticulous and comprehensive entity extraction in medical texts, providing stronger support for digging into medical information.

4 Experiment

4.1 Experimental Setting

Experimental Parameters Setting: The experiment uses the BERT-based model as the backbone of the experiment and ChatGLM3.0 as the main model for entity extraction. The model is built under the Pytorch framework. The parameters of the BERT model are set as follows: the Adam is selected as the optimiser, the learning rate is set to $1e-4$, the batch size is set to 8, the hidden variables are set to 1024, and the dropout is set to 0.5 in order to prevent overfitting, and the ChatGLM is fine-tuned by using P-turning.

4.2 Experimental Results

In the experiment, abstract training was conducted for 2 rounds, and the best F1 submitted was 0.2417 (total 0.25). Since the title was divided into two parts, in order to ensure accurate F1 value calculation, we combined them into a complete title for submission. The title classification part was trained for 2 rounds, and the title information extraction part was trained for 30 rounds. After submission testing, the 25th round had the best effect, with the best F1 of 0.5561 (total 0.75), so the total score was 0.7978.

5 Conclusion

Based on the CHIP2023-PICOS evaluation task, this article explores the differences between traditional pre-training models and big models in information extraction tasks. It was found that traditional pre-training models still outperform big models in classification tasks, so the information extraction task was detailed and split into two subtasks: classification and information extraction, in order to achieve better results. Our research results show that big models achieve higher accuracy when training multiple tasks at the same time, possibly because there are more tasks and the amount of useful knowledge that can be learned between tasks increases, and the increase in data brings strong generalization. However, in simple classification tasks, big models are not as effective as pre-trained models. This may be because the features constructed by big models are more complex and consider more factors, but more information features in simple tasks may be a burden on feature engineering. Finally, we combined the comprehensive results of the subtasks. In evaluation test B, the results of title information extraction and abstract classification were 0.2417 and 0.5561, respectively. The final result was 0.7978, ranking second in terms of open-source code.

References

1. Labrak, Y., Rouvier, M., Dufour, R.: A zero-shot and few-shot study of instruction-finetuned large language models applied to clinical and biomedical tasks. arXiv (2023). http://arxiv.org/abs/2307.12114, https://doi.org/10.48550/arXiv.2307.12114. Accessed 20 Oct 2023
2. Gao, J., Zhao, H., Yu, C.: Exploring the feasibility of ChatGPT for event extraction. arXiv (2023). http://arxiv.org/abs/2303.03836, https://doi.org/10.48550/arXiv.2303.03836. Accessed 01 Nov 2023
3. Vaswani, A., Shazeer, N., Parmar, N.: Attention is all you need. arXiv (2017). http://arxiv.org/abs/1706.03762. Accessed 08 June 2023
4. Brown, T.B., Mann, B., Ryder, N.: Language models are few-shot learners. arXiv (2020). http://arxiv.org/abs/2005.14165, https://doi.org/10.48550/arXiv.2005.14165. Accessed 07 Oct 2023
5. Chang, Y., Wang, X., Wang, J.: A survey on evaluation of large language models. arXiv (2023). http://arxiv.org/abs/2307.03109, https://doi.org/10.48550/arXiv.2307.03109. Accessed 03 Oct 2023
6. Wei, J., Tay, Y., Bommasani, R.: Emergent abilities of large language models. arXiv (2022). http://arxiv.org/abs/2206.07682, https://doi.org/10.48550/arXiv.2206.07682. Accessed 06 Oct 2023
7. Han, R., Peng, T., Yang, C.: Is information extraction solved by ChatGPT? An analysis of performance, evaluation criteria, robustness and errors (2023). https://arxiv.org/abs/2305.14450v1. Accessed 29 Oct 2023
8. Devlin, J., Chang, M.W., Lee, K.: BERT: pre-training of deep bidirectional transformers for language understanding. arXiv (2019). http://arxiv.org/abs/1810.04805. Accessed 08 June 2023
9. Wang, Y., Wang, L., Rastegar-Mojarad, M.: Clinical information extraction applications: a literature review. J. Biomed. Inform. 77, 34–49 (2018). https://doi.org/10.1016/j.jbi.2017.11.011
10. Global Context-enhanced Graph Convolutional Networks for Document-level Relation Extraction - ACL Anthology (2024). https://aclanthology.org/2020.coling-main.461/
11. Ren, F., Zhang, L., Yin, S., et al.: A novel global f-eature-oriented relational triple extraction model based on table filling. In: Proceedings of the 2021 Conference on Empirical Methods in Natural Language Processing, pp. 2646–2656. Association for Computational Linguistics, Online and Punta Cana (2021)
12. Miwa, M., Bansal, M.: End-to-end relation extraction using LSTMs on sequences and tree structures. In: Proceedings of the 54th Annual Meeting of the Association for Computational Linguistics (Volume 1: Long Papers), pp. 1105–1116. Association for Computational Linguistics, Berlin (2016)

13. Yan, Z., Zhang, C., Fu, J., et al.: A partition filter network for joint entity and relation extraction. In: Proceedings of the 2021 Conference on Empirical Methods in Natural Language Processing, pp. 185–197. Association for Computational Linguistics, Online and Punta Cana (2021)

14. Xu, N., Xie, H., Zhao, D.: A novel joint framework for multiple Chinese events extraction. In: Sun, M., Li, S., Zhang, Y., Liu, Y., He, S., Rao, G. (eds.) CCL 2020. LNCS, vol. 12522, pp. 174–183. Springer, Cham (2020). https://doi.org/10.1007/978-3-030-63031-7_13

15. 冯兴杰, 赵新阳冯小荣: 基于软参数共享的事件联合抽取方法. 计算机应用研究 **40**(1), 91–96 (2023)

16. Abdullah, M.H.A., Aziz, N., Abdulkadir S.J.: Systematic literature review of information extraction from textual data: recent methods, applications, trends, and challenges. IEEE Access **11**, 10535–10562 (2023). https://doi.org/10.1109/ACCESS.2023.3240898

17. Zhong, Z., Chen, D.: A frustratingly easy approach for entity and relation extraction. In: Proceedings of the 2021 Conference of the North American Chapter of the Association for Computational Linguistics: Human Language Technologies, pp. 50–61. Association for Computational Linguistics (2021)

18. Xiong, X., Yunfei, L., Anqi, L., et al.: A multi-gate encoder for joint entity and relation extraction. In: Proceedings of the 21st Chinese National Conference on Computational Linguistics, pp. 848–860. Chinese Information Processing Society of China, Nanchang (2022)

19. Lu, Y., Liu, Q., Dai, D.: Unified structure generation for universal information extraction. In: Proceedings of the 60th Annual Meeting of the Association for Computational Linguistics (Volume 1: Long Papers), pp. 5755–5772. Association for Computational Linguistics, Dublin (2022). https://aclanthology.org/2022.acl-long.395, https://doi.org/10.18653/v1/2022.acl-long.395

20. Wei, X., Cui, X., Cheng, N.: Zero-shot information extraction via chatting with ChatGPT. (2023). https://arxiv.org/abs/2302.10205v1. Accessed 30 Oct 2023

21. Madry, A., Makelov, A., Schmidt, L.: Towards deep learning models resistant to adversarial attacks. arXiv (2019). http://arxiv.org/abs/1706.06083, https://doi.org/10.48550/arXiv.1706.06083. Accessed 10 Dec 2023

22. Liu, Y., Ott, M., Goyal, N.: RoBERTa: a robustly optimized BERT pretraining approach. arXiv (2019). http://arxiv.org/abs/1907.11692, https://doi.org/10.48550/arXiv.1907.11692. Accessed 10 Dec 2023

23. Du, Z., Qian, Y., Liu, X.: GLM: general language model pretraining with autoregressive blank infilling. arXiv (2022). http://arxiv.org/abs/2103.10360, https://doi.org/10.48550/arXiv.2103.10360. Accessed 10 Dec 2023

24. Liu, X., Zheng, Y., Du, Z.: GPT understands, too. arXiv (2023). http://arxiv.org/abs/2103.10385, https://doi.org/10.48550/arXiv.2103.10385. Accessed 10 Dec 2023

Enhancing PICOS Information Extraction with UIE and ERNIE-Health

Lei Zhang, Wei Tian$^{(\boxtimes)}$, Yuan Zheng, and Yue Jian

Beijing Smartdot Technology Co., Ltd., Beijing 100080, China
tianwei@smartdot.com

Abstract. In the vast sea of medical papers lie numerous crucial pieces of information. Faced with the challenge of unstructured medical literature, it becomes a formidable task to automatically extract the necessary key information. In this paper, we delve into the CHIP2023 evaluation task 5, utilizing UIE and ERNIE-Health to accomplish the extraction of PICOS key information from medical papers. Our results indicate that the framework we propose has achieved commendable performance.

Keywords: UIE · ERNIE-Health · PICOS

1 Introduction

In today's field of medical research, with the continuous advancement of technology and the extensive expansion of studies, a vast amount of literature has become a crucial source for researchers to acquire new knowledge and conduct comprehensive analyses. However, the subsequent challenge is how to efficiently and accurately retrieve and categorize this literature to meet the diverse needs of researchers in various fields-a primary concern in the current landscape. Particularly in medical research, due to the diversity in research designs and objectives, traditional retrieval methods and classification tools often struggle to adequately fulfill this task.

The PICOS principle, serving as a standardized framework for designing medical research, offers a systematic approach to define the key elements of a study. Nevertheless, in practical academic searches, researchers still face the challenge of accurately extracting and understanding PICOS elements from a vast amount of literature. Additionally, existing keyword retrieval methods, while convenient, often fall short in fully considering the diversity of literature and the complexity of information.

The traditional keyword retrieval method may not adequately capture the hidden PICOS elements in literature, especially as research questions and methods become more complex. Researchers may face diverse expressions and terms in the literature, leading to potential omissions or misunderstandings during the information extraction process. Additionally, certain key information may appear in different forms, increasing the difficulty for researchers to accurately locate these elements in the literature.

© The Author(s), under exclusive license to Springer Nature Singapore Pte Ltd. 2024
H. Xu et al. (Eds.): CHIP 2023, CCIS 2080, pp. 186–194, 2024.
https://doi.org/10.1007/978-981-97-1717-0_17

Therefore, it is essential to explore more advanced, intelligent information extraction techniques to assist researchers in accurately extracting and understanding PICOS elements from literature. This may involve natural language processing techniques, information extraction algorithms, or even models based on deep learning to comprehensively and precisely capture key information in the literature. Through such approaches, researchers can more efficiently utilize the PICOS principles, promoting the quality and accuracy of medical research design and literature reviews.

The competition task has defined two distinct objectives based on the practical requirements. These objectives involve extracting decision-related information from paper titles and identifying the intent of different sentences within paper abstracts. To address this issue, we propose an innovative approach that comprehensively applies UIE [1] and ERNIE-Health [2]. Utilizing ERNIE-Health, pretrained on medical texts, for the intent recognition task, and employing UIE for the decision-related information extraction task.

2   Related Work

In the field of medical literature processing, research has consistently focused on information extraction and text classification. Entity extraction in information extraction aims to extract crucial entities from intricate medical texts, while text classification is dedicated to efficiently assigning literature content to various categories. Scholars in past research have made significant advancements by employing a variety of techniques and methods, including rule-based systems, machine learning algorithms, and more recently, deep learning models.

2.1   Information Extraction-Related Tasks

Information extraction, as a crucial task in the field of natural language processing, is dedicated to automatically extracting structured information from text. In recent years, with the rise of deep learning and pre-trained models, the field of information extraction has undergone significant development, providing more powerful tools for handling the context and semantic relationships of natural language.

Traditional information extraction methods mainly include rule-based methods and statistical-based methods. Rule-based methods extract entities and relationships using predefined rules, such as regular expressions or manually constructed rules. However, these methods are often limited by the coverage and flexibility of the rules, making it challenging to adapt to the diversity of terms and complexity of context in medical literature.

With the introduction of statistical learning methods such as Conditional Random Fields and Maximum Entropy Models [3], there have been some advancements in information extraction. However, manual feature design is still required, limiting its adaptability. With the rise of deep learning technologies, models like Recurrent Neural Networks (RNNs) [4] and Long Short-Term Memory Networks (LSTMs) [5] have been introduced to information extraction tasks. These models can learn long-term dependencies in context. However, in fields like medical literature, they may encounter challenges such as data scarcity and label noise due to the complexity of the data.

Yaojie Lu and colleagues proposed the Universal Information Extraction (UIE) framework at ACL-2022. This framework achieves a unified modeling of tasks such as entity extraction, relation extraction, event extraction, and sentiment analysis. It endows different tasks with strong transfer and generalization capabilities. Utilizing the knowledge-enhanced pre-training model ERNIE 3.0 [6], they trained and open-sourced the first Chinese universal information extraction model, UIE. This model supports key information extraction without constraints on industry domains and extraction targets. It enables zero-shot rapid cold start and exhibits excellent fine-tuning capabilities for small samples, quickly adapting to specific extraction goals.

In our research, we leverage the UIE technology and incorporate adversarial training to extract key information regarding the PICOS principles from medical literature. This approach allows us to better adapt to the diversity of medical literature, enhancing the accuracy and comprehensiveness of information extraction.

2.2   Text Classification-Related Work

Text classification is a crucial task in natural language processing, aiming to assign given text to predefined categories. This task is prevalent in many application scenarios, such as medical text classification, sentiment analysis, news categorization, and more.

Traditional text classification methods mainly include statistical-based approaches such as the bag-of-words model and TF-IDF [7]. These methods overlook the semantic relationships between words, making it challenging to capture deep semantic information in the text. In the medical field, such approaches may struggle to understand specialized terminology and context effectively.

With the rise of deep learning, especially Convolutional Neural Networks [8] and Recurrent Neural Networks (RNNs), text classification has made significant progress. Deep learning models can automatically learn richer, high-level feature representations, thereby better capturing the semantic information in the text. BERT (Bidirectional Encoder Representations from Transformers) [9] is a pre-trained model based on the Transformer architecture, introduced by Google in 2018. Its uniqueness lies in bidirectional context modeling, enabling a more comprehensive understanding of context and capturing complex relationships between vocabulary. Following BERT's success, various improvements and variants have emerged. For instance, RoBERTa [10] enhances performance through hyperparameter tuning and longer training sentences, DistillBERT [11] compresses the model through distillation methods for improved efficiency, and ALBERT [12] reduces the number of parameters through parameter sharing and cross-layer parameter connections. XLNet [13] combines autoregressive and autoencoding principles, ERNIE [14] introduces knowledge enhancement, and MACBERT [15] enhances the model's adaptability to context across different tasks through meta-learning mechanisms. These variants demonstrate outstanding performance in their respective fields and tasks. ERNIE-Health, on the other hand, is a product of further pre-training in the medical domain, focusing on understanding the specificity of medical texts. Models of this kind have achieved significant success in tasks such as medical literature classification.

In our research, we incorporate ERNIE-Health into text classification tasks to enhance the understanding and categorization of medical literature. We conducted in-depth exploration specifically addressing the multi-label classification challenge in literature. By employing a fine-grained label system, we aim to classify literature more comprehensively and accurately, capturing its diverse nature.

By integrating UIE technology and ERNIE-Health, our research aims to address key challenges in information extraction and text classification in handling medical literature. We aspire to provide medical researchers with more precise and comprehensive tools for understanding and retrieving literature.

3   Proposed Framework

In our research, the proposed framework integrates UIE (information extraction) and the ERNIE-Health model, aiming to accomplish the task of extracting PICOS key information from medical literature. We fine-tune the UIE model based on provided medical data for training, enabling the extraction of critical information from literature, covering elements of the PICOS principles such as the study population, intervention, comparison, outcomes, and study design types. On the other hand, we fine-tune the ERNIE-Health model based on the provided training set to achieve a deep understanding of literature and precise classification.

3.1   Main Model

In our medical paper PICOS key information extraction task, we implemented a series of impactful strategies to enhance the model's performance and robustness. Firstly, the UIE-medical model was introduced to specifically tackle the complexity of medical literature, successfully achieving the extraction of PICOS key information. To bolster the model's robustness, we introduced FGM [16], an adversarial training method that introduces small but targeted perturbations to the input during training, enhancing the model's adaptability to adversarial perturbations and better capturing crucial information in the text.

For classification tasks, we introduced the ERNIE-Health pre-trained model, leveraging its rich understanding of the medical domain. Combining FGM and k-fold cross-validation, our aim was to improve the model's generalization performance, ensuring robustness across different domains and data distributions. This deeply integrated approach not only considers the precision of information extraction but also emphasizes the model's adaptability to medical contexts and diverse data.

In summary, our comprehensive approach not only focuses on the core task of PICOS key information extraction but also provides a holistic and powerful solution for medical literature classification tasks, as illustrated in (see Fig. 1).

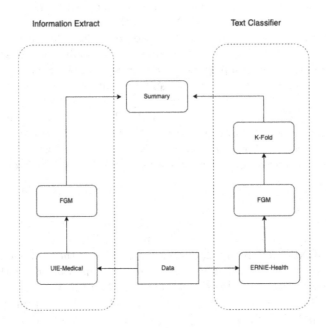

Fig. 1. The architecture diagram for the PICOS key information extraction task.

Information extraction suffers from its varying targets, heterogeneous structures, and demand-specific schemas. The unified text-to-structure generation framework, namely UIE, can universally model different IE tasks, adaptively generate targeted structures, and collaboratively learn general IE abilities from different knowledge sources. Specifically, UIE uniformly encodes different extraction structures via a structured extraction language, adaptively generates target extractions via a schema-based prompt mechanism - structural schema instructor, and captures the common IE abilities via a large-scale pre-trained text-to-structure model (see Fig. 2).

To adapt to key information extraction in medical papers, we conducted fine-tuning on the UIE model using annotated data, specifically tailored for the entity extraction task in medical literature.

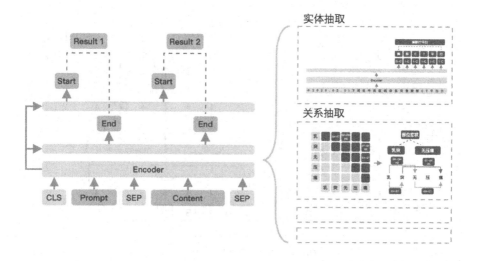

Fig. 2. Main structure of UIE model.

To cater to the extraction of crucial information in medical papers, ERNIE-Health is built on Baidu's advanced knowledge-enhanced pre-trained language model, ERNIE. Through the application of medical knowledge enhancement techniques, it further learns from vast amounts of medical data, accurately grasping professional medical knowledge. ERNIE-Health utilizes medical entity masking strategies, concentrating on learning entity-level knowledge such as professional terms, acquiring a comprehensive understanding of diverse medical entities. Concurrently, by engaging in tasks like medical question matching, it learns the correlation between patient symptom descriptions and doctors' specialized treatment plans, deepening its grasp of intrinsic connections within medical entity knowledge. ERNIE-Health has undergone training with over 600,000 medical professional terms and more than 40 million medical professional terms, significantly boosting its comprehension and modeling capabilities of medical expertise. Additionally, ERNIE-Health explores multi-level semantic discrimination pre-training tasks, enhancing the model's efficiency in acquiring medical knowledge. The overall structure of this model bears similarity to ELECTRA, consisting of generator and discriminator components (see Fig. 3).

To tailor ERNIE-Health for key information extaction in medical papers, we conducted fine-tuning using annotated data. This fine-tuning specifically aimed at adapting the ERNIE-Health model for the task of sentence classification in medical literature.

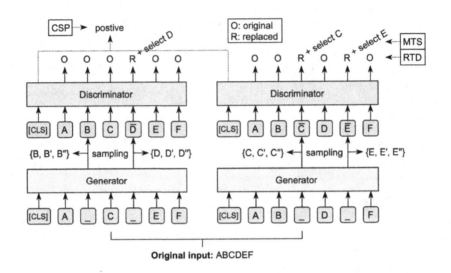

Fig. 3. Main structure of ERNIE-Health model.

4   Experiment

4.1   Datasets

The task involves extracting key information from medical papers, and the data is divided into training, validation, and test sets, totaling 4,500 entries. The dataset is stored in JSON format. Specifically, the training set comprises 2,000 entries, the validation set consists of 500 entries, and the test set comprises 2,000 entries.

4.2   Information Extraction

In our research, we employed UIE for performing medical text information extraction tasks. Through domain fine-tuning on the training data, we successfully enhanced the model's adaptability to the medical domain. In the inference phase, to further optimize performance, we mitigated the risk of false recall by setting a threshold. For entities extracted by the UIE model, we apply a threshold treatment by setting the probability value for entities to 0.59, and through experimentation with multiple thresholds, we found that at this threshold, the F1 score for the information extraction task reached its highest level. The successful application of this strategy resulted in our model achieving outstanding performance in information extraction tasks, accurately capturing crucial information in medical texts.

4.3 Text Classification

During our research phase, we chose to fine-tune with ERNIE-Health to better adapt to the context of the medical domain. Employing a strategy of 5-fold cross-validation, we generated five independent models on the training set. In each fold, we fine-tuned the model to ensure robust performance across different subsets of training data.

To integrate the predictions of multiple models, we used a voting mechanism. Specifically, each model made predictions on the test samples, and we counted the votes for each category. In the end, the label with the highest number of votes was selected as the final label for that sample. This voting mechanism helps alleviate errors that may arise from a single model, enhancing the overall robustness and accuracy of the model.

With this research strategy, our goal was to fully leverage the pre-training capabilities of ERNIE-Health, refine it through fine-tuning to better suit the context of the medical domain, and improve the stability and performance of classification through multi-model voting.

4.4 Setting

Both UIE and Ernie-Heath utilize AdamW as the optimizer with cosine decay. The learning rate for UIE is set at $2e-5$, while Ernie-Health uses a learning rate of $1e-5$. UIE is trained for 20 epochs, whereas ERNIE-Health undergoes 10 epochs. Both models are built using Transformers 4.7.0 and PyTorch 1.10.1 for training.

4.5 Experimental Results

To facilitate a comprehensive comparison, we compared four selected approaches: UIE-base+BERT, UIE-base+ERNIE-Health, UIE-medical+ERNIE-Health, and UIE-medical+ERNIE-Health+FGM. UIE and ERNIE, pre-trained on medical texts, exhibited superior performance in the extraction of PICOS key information from medical papers. Finally, FGM was introduced to enhance the model's robustness. The comparative results are presented in Table 1.

Table 1. The score evaluation results of TestB in CHIP2023 Evaluation 5.

Model	Score(F1)
UIE-base+BERT	0.7802
UIE-base+ERNIE-Health	0.7856
UIE-medical+ERNIE-Health	0.7910
UIE-medical+ERNIE-Health+FGM	0.7962

5   Conclusion

This paper is based on the CHIP 2023 evaluation task 5. We jointly leverage UIE and Ernie-Health to accomplish the extraction of PICOS key information in medical papers. To enhance results, we conduct domain fine-tuning based on the UIE model. During the inference stage, we set a threshold of 0.59 to reduce false recalls in the information extraction task. On the other hand, using Ernie-Health, we tackle the sentence classification task and employ a five-fold cross-validation approach to enhance model robustness. Ultimately, we achieve a score of 0.7962, securing the third position in the open-source code rankings.

References

1. Lu, Y., Liu, Q., Dai, D., et al.: Unified structure generation for universal information extraction. arXiv preprint arXiv:2203.12277 (2022)
2. Wang, Q., Dai, S., Xu, B., et al.: Building Chinese biomedical language models via multi-level text discrimination. arXiv preprint arXiv:2110.07244 (2021)
3. Baldwin, R.A.: Use of maximum entropy modeling in wildlife research. Entropy 11(4), 854–866 (2009)
4. Grossberg, S.: Recurrent neural networks. Scholarpedia 8(2), 1888 (2013)
5. Cheng, J., Dong, L., Lapata, M.: Long short-term memory-networks for machine reading. arXiv preprint arXiv:1601.06733 (2016)
6. Sun, Y., Wang, S., Feng, S., et al.: ERNIE 3.0: large-scale knowledge enhanced pre-training for language understanding and generation. arXiv preprint arXiv:2107.02137 (2021)
7. Qaiser, S., Ali, R.: Text mining: use of TF-IDF to examine the relevance of words to documents. Int. J. Comput. Appl. 181(1), 25–29 (2018)
8. Li, Z., Liu, F., Yang, W., et al.: A survey of convolutional neural networks: analysis, applications, and prospects. IEEE Trans. Neural Netw. Learn. Syst. (2021)
9. Devlin, J., Chang, M.W., Lee, K., et al.: BERT: pre-training of deep bidirectional transformers for language understanding. arXiv preprint arXiv:1810.04805 (2018)
10. Liu, Y., Ott, M., Goyal, N., et al.: RoBERTa: a robustly optimized BERT pre-training approach. arXiv preprint arXiv:1907.11692 (2019)
11. Sanh, V., Debut, L., Chaumond, J., et al.: DistilBERT, a distilled version of BERT: smaller, faster, cheaper and lighter. arXiv preprint arXiv:1910.01108 (2019)
12. Lan, Z., Chen, M., Goodman, S., et al.: AlBERT: a lite BERT for self-supervised learning of language representations. arXiv preprint arXiv:1909.11942 (2019)
13. Yang, Z., Dai, Z., Yang, Y., et al.: XLNet: generalized autoregressive pretraining for language understanding. In: Advances in Neural Information Processing Systems, vol. 32 (2019)
14. Sun, Y., Wang, S., Li, Y., et al.: ERNIE: enhanced representation through knowledge integration. arXiv preprint arXiv:1904.09223 (2019)
15. Cui, Y., Che, W., Liu, T., et al.: Revisiting pre-trained models for Chinese natural language processing. arXiv preprint arXiv:2004.13922 (2020)
16. Miyato, T., Dai, A.M., Goodfellow, I.: Adversarial training methods for semi-supervised text classification. arXiv preprint arXiv:1605.07725 (2016)

Chinese Diabetes Question Classification

The CHIP 2023 Shared Task 6: Chinese Diabetes Question Classification

Shunhao Li[1], Xiaobo Qian[1], Kehui Tan[1,2], Maojie Wang[3,4,5], and Tianyong Hao[1(✉)]

[1] School of Computer Science, South China Normal University, Guangzhou, China
lishunhao99@foxmail.com, xiaoboqian1221@outlook.com,
kehui.tt@gmail.com, haoty@m.scnu.edu.cn
[2] School of Artificial Intelligence, South China Normal University, Guangzhou, China
[3] The Second Affiliated Hospital of Guangzhou University of Chinese Medicine (Guangdong Provincial Hospital of Chinese Medicine), Guangzhou, China
maojiewang@gzucm.edu.cn
[4] Guangdong Provincial Key Laboratory of Clinical Research On Traditional Chinese Medicine Syndrome, Guangzhou, China
[5] State Key Laboratory of Dampness Syndrome of Chinese Medicine, The Second Affiliated Hospital of Guangzhou University of Chinese Medicine, Guangzhou, China

Abstract. Medical question classification is one of essential tasks in the processing of medical question data for enhancing the capability of medical automatic question answering systems. However, the unique characteristics of medical questions, such as the abundance of uncommon medical terms and the presence of ambiguous short texts, result in challenges to obtain the most essential information of user intents. The primary focus of this shared task is the classification of Chinese diabetes questions from patient users. The shared task was organized in an international conference CHIP 2023 and attracted anticipations of more than 20 teams from both industry and academia. Top three of these participants showed promising performance. This paper provides a concise overview and summary of the various approaches explored by the participating teams during the competition.

Keywords: Question Classification · Diabetes · Medical data processing

1 Introduction

With the rapid development of the Internet, there is an increasing demand among a vast population of individuals with diabetes for accessing professional information about diabetes. The importance of automatic question answering services for diabetic patients is continuously growing as it meets the daily health service needs of the patients and high-risk individuals. The Chinese diabetes question classification evaluation task aims to automatically classify diabetes-related questions posed by patients, enhance search performance, and drive the development of automatic question answering services for diabetic patients [1, 2]. Accurate classification and understanding of diabetes question can provide precise information and guidance to healthcare professionals and patients

[3], thereby promoting the management and prevention of diabetes disease. Therefore, research on Chinese diabetes question classification holds significant practical significance and application potential.

Diabetes is a common chronic disease that significantly affects patients' quality of life and health. With the increasing pace of life and changes in dietary habits, the incidence of diabetes continues to rise [4]. In this context, a diabetes automatic question answering system can meet people's needs for obtaining diabetes information. It can provide accurate and reliable information, answer users' questions, and offer personalized suggestions, such as dietary guidance and medication usage tips, etc. The field of diabetes encompasses various question types, including symptoms, diagnosis, treatment, and lifestyle, which makes question classification complex. Therefore, enabling systems to accurately understand and classify problems into corresponding categories remains an urgent issue.

The Chinese diabetes question classification evaluation task aims to automatically classify diabetes-related questions posed by patients. This task contributes to improving the performance of search results and driving the development of automatic question-answering services for diabetes. Participants are required to predict the categories corresponding to the diabetes questions and fill in the missing category labels in the test dataset. The evaluation phase analyzes the errors in the filled-in data to obtain the performance score. In this task, we use the diabetes benchmark dataset proposed by Qian et al. [5] as the evaluation dataset. This task attracted participations from both industry and academia, with the top three teams achieving scores of 92.1%, 92.0%, and 90.7% respectively. Section 3 describes the dataset, including dataset collection, statistics, evaluation metrics, and baselines. The baseline results are described in Sect. 4.1, while the results of the methods by participating teams are provided in Sect. 4.2.

2   Related Work

The China Health Information Processing Conference (CHIP2023) is a significant academic conference organized by the Medical Health and Bioinformatics Processing Committee of the China Information Processing Society (CIPS). It aims to promote research and application in the field of health information processing. As a prominent conference in the field of health information processing in China, it provides a platform for researchers and practitioners from academia and industry to exchange ideas, share research results, and showcase experiences. The theme of the 2023 conference is "Large Models and Intelligent Healthcare," focusing on the trends and challenges of intelligent healthcare development in the era of large models. The conference brings together leading medical information processing scholars and healthcare experts from across the country to explore new avenues for applying artificial intelligence in healthcare and innovative methods for medical research. Participation in such a conference allows researchers and practitioners to share their latest research findings, exchange ideas, and explore collaboration opportunities, thereby fostering innovation and development in the field of intelligent healthcare. This conference plays a significant role in advancing cutting-edge research in medical and health information processing and promoting the application and implementation of related technologies.

Text Classification (TC) is one of the fundamental tasks in Natural Language Processing (NLP). With the widespread application of deep learning in NLP, TC technology has made significant advancements. Early Recurrent Neural Networks (RNNs) like LSTM [6] captured cross-temporal patterns within sequences for classification, but their computational cost increased significantly with longer sequences. Convolutional Neural Networks (CNNs) learned local contextual relationships between adjacent words or features, such as DCNN [7], but struggled to capture global sequence information effectively. Subsequently, researchers began incorporating Graph Neural Network (GNN) concepts, treating text as a complex relational network, such as syntactic or semantic parsing trees. Early GNN models such as TextRank [8] excelled at capturing relationships between words or phrases of different types, such as vocabulary or semantics, laying the foundation for capturing global text features. The Transformer [9] architecture simulated the influence of words on the overall sequence using self-attention mechanisms, enabling efficient parallel computation. It overcame the computational limitations of RNNs while incorporating the strengths of RNNs and CNNs. Memory networks, such as NSE [10], introduced external writable memory, enabling models to retrieve more widely relevant information from broader knowledge compared to attention models with more scalable memory. Recently, large-scale Pre-trained Language Models (PLMs) like GPT-4 and Claude achieved breakthroughs by pre-training on extensive corpora in an unsupervised manner and fine-tuning on downstream tasks. This demonstrated the broad application prospects of the pre-training fine-tuning framework in NLP tasks.

Some research efforts have been made by domestic and international scholars on the construction of medical question taxonomies. Representative classification systems include the TGCQ [11] clinical question classification and ICPC-2 [12] for primary medical care classification. However, these systems were developed based on physicians' information needs and not directly suitable for expressing patients' intentions or classifying users' health issues. In recent years, some studies have proposed intention-oriented question classification systems for specific medical domains such as cancer [13], genetic diseases [14] and diabetes [15]. However, these systems are limited to coarse-grained classifications and lack fine-grained classification capabilities.

The development of Chinese medical question corpora has been relatively recent. Guo [16] constructed a classification corpus specially for common medical interview questions related to diabetes. However, this corpus primarily focuses on medical characteristics while neglecting users' health information needs. Therefore, there is a need for a diabetes automatic question answering system that can provide personalized information services to diabetic patients and individuals at high risk. By classifying Chinese diabetes questions, the system can offer tailored recommendations, guidance, and answers based on different question types to meet their specific needs for diabetes-related information.

3 Dataset

3.1 Dataset Collection

The dataset used in this shared task was collected from two major medical question and answer websites in China: "39 Health" and "Have Question Must Answer". On these sites, every posed question received answers from professional clinicians working in domestic hospitals. We considered the original user questions and the corresponding replies from clinicians as the raw data for our study. Following the cleaning and pre-processing of the collected raw data, we created a question-answer corpus. To create an annotated dataset specifically for diabetes questions, we randomly sampled 8,000 questions to conduct manual annotation. Initially, one annotator with a medical informatics background annotated all 8,000 diabetes questions in the dataset. Additionally, two more annotators each annotated 1,000 questions randomly sampled from the all 8,000 questions. After the initial annotation, we assessed the consistency of annotations among the three annotators and discussed discrepancies to reach a consensus. We then updated the annotation schema and guidelines accordingly. Subsequently, the three annotators inde-pendently re-annotated the remaining 6,000 questions following the modified annotation guidelines, with each annotating 2,000 questions. Finally, we compared the annotation results from the three annotators, discussed discrepancies that arose during the anno-tation process to reach a consensus, and further revised and finalized the annotation guidelines.

To evaluate the consistency and quality of dataset annotation, it is necessary to identify divergences between the annotators. We use the Kappa statistic to assess the Inter Annotator Agreement (IAA), which measures the level of agreement among the annotators. Kappa, a widely applied metric for IAA [17], quantifies the agreement beyond what would be expected by chance. The calculation of Kappa is shown in Eq. (1).

$$Kappa = \frac{(P_o - P_e)}{(1 - P_e)}, \tag{1}$$

P_o is the overall classification accuracy, which is the sum of correct classifications in each category divided by the total number of samples, and P_e is accidental consistency [18]. A higher Kappa value indicates better annotation consistency. In this study, if the annotators annotate the same main category and fine-grained category, it is considered an agreement. Throughout the annotation process, the average annotation consistency among the three annotators was 0.78, indicating minimal differences in manual anno-tations and suggesting that the established classification system was reasonable and effective.

3.2 Dataset Statistics

The dataset used in this shared task consisted of 8,000 Chinese diabetes questions, which were categorized into six categories: diagnosis, treatment, common knowledge, healthy lifestyle, epidemiology, and other. Each medical question text was labeled with two components: "questions" and "label". Among the questions, 6,000 were used for model training, 1,000 for validation, and 1,000 for testing. Participants were required to predict the corresponding category of diabetes questions in the test set based on the content of the "question" component. Table 1 shows the statistics of the task dataset.

Table 1. The statistics of the dataset used in the shared task.

Categories	Training Set	Validation Set	Test Set	Total
Diagnosis	527	103	87	717
Treatment	1,501	260	265	2,026
Common Knowledge	1,226	212	217	1,655
Healthy Lifestyle	1,702	251	273	2,226
Epidemiology	599	118	90	807
Other	445	56	68	569
Total	6,000	1,000	1,000	8,000

3.3 Evaluation

The task used accuracy (ACC) as an evaluation metrics. Accuracy is a widely used evaluation metric in machine learning and classification tasks. It measures the proportion of correctly classified instances or samples in a dataset. The accuracy is described below:

$$ACC = \frac{TP}{TP + FP}, \tag{2}$$

where TP is True Positive and FP is False Positive. ACC is defined as the number of correct predictions made by the model divided by the total number of predictions, which includes TP and FP. Precision measures the accuracy of the model and can provide an intuitive assessment of its quality.

3.4 Baseline Models

Three baseline models were applied for testing on the Chinese diabetes question dataset, i.e., Text Convolutional Neural Network (Text CNN), Text Recurrent Neural Network (Text RNN), and Bidirectional Encoder Representation from Transformer model (BERT).

Text CNN: Kim [7] introduced the Text CNN model for text classification tasks, harnessing the power of CNN to capture local features in input text. It utilized convolutional layers to extract text features and employs multiple convolutional kernels to capture features of various lengths. These extracted features were then mapped to different classification labels through fully connected layers, enabling CNN to excel in natural language processing problem classification tasks. With thoughtful model design and hyperparameter tuning, CNN had demonstrated the capability to achieve high accuracy and robustness in such tasks.

Text RNN: CNN demonstrated potential in classification tasks but it had certain drawbacks. CNN was not well-suited for handling variable-length sequence data or capturing contextual information in text, leading to a loss of crucial semantic information in specific tasks. Addressing these limitations, Liu [19] proposed Text RNN in 2016. Text RNN treated text as a sequence and learned sequence information by passing hidden states at each time step. Consequently, Text RNN was adept at handling variable-length sequence data and capturing contextual information in text.

BERT: The Google research team introduced BERT, a pre-trained language model derived from the Transformer architecture [20]. BERT leveraged the self-attention mechanism, enabling it to attend to different positions in the input sequence simultaneously and model contextual information. Demonstrating exceptional performance in handling long sequences and capturing long-term dependencies, BERT had undergone pre-training and fine-tuning on specific tasks, achieving remarkable improvements in various natural language processing tasks, including text classification.

4   The Results

4.1   Overall Statistics

The shared task received a total of 116 submissions from participating teams. The maximum accuracy achieved was 92.1%, the minimum accuracy was 21.8%, the average accuracy across all submissions was 87.6%, with a median accuracy of 89.0%. The standard deviation of accuracy was 7.78. The statistical results are presented in Table 2.

Table 2. Overall statistics of accuracy performance from all teams.

Number of Teams	Max (%)	Min (%)	Average (%)	Median (%)	Standard deviation
116	92.1	21.8	87.6	89.0	7.78

4.2   Top-3 Performance

Table 3 displays the accuracy results of the baseline methods and the top three teams. Baseline 1, Baseline 2, and Baseline 3 utilized Text CNN, Text RNN, and BERT as methods, achieving accuracy of 86.1%, 83.8%, and 87.8%, respectively. The first and second ranking teams used baichuan2-13b and Qwen-7b+claude2 as methods, attaining accuracy of 92.1% and 92.0%, respectively. The third ranking team utilized a hybrid method of BERT and voting strategy, achieving an accuracy of 90.7%.

The first team devised an innovative workflow to address the task of diabetes question classification. The team transformed the text classification problem into a text generation task through prompt construction, minimizing results outside the specified categories. To enhance the accuracy of classification, they employed the LoRA method to fine-tune the large language model. Additionally, to enhance the capability in the medical domain, they employed another open-source dataset for initial fine-tuning of the model, followed by transfer learning to fine-tune the Chinese diabetes questions dataset.

The second team proposed a model integration approach for this task, combining small models with large pre-trained language models to address the misclassification situation of single-model classification by leveraging the respective advantages of large

Table 3. The scores of baseline methods and the top three teams.

Teams	Methods	ACC (%)
Baseline 1	Text CNN	86.1
Baseline 2	Text RNN	83.8
Baseline 3	BERT	87.8
Team 1 (hmkj)	baichuan2-13b	92.1
Team 2 (少喝奶茶受益终生)	Qwen-7b + claude2	92.0
Team 3 (zzu_nlp_炼药师)	BERT + voting	90.7

and small models. To continuously optimize the model, the team employed external tools to expand the number of challenging samples. They then utilized a voting mechanism, where the results of multiple model classifications were aggregated through voting. The output with the highest number of votes was considered the final prediction using a majority voting strategy.

The third team employed a multi-language back-translation strategy combined with sentence vector similarity comparison to enhance the training set. They utilized the bge-large-zh-v1.5 semantic vector model to generate sentence vectors. A cosine similarity comparison between sentence vectors was conducted to filter back-translated samples, leading to an improvement in the quality of the augmented data. Additionally, the team introduced a model ensemble approach, aggregating predictions from various models through second-level voting. This ensemble strategy demonstrated significant improvements compared to individual models.

5   Conclusion

This paper introduced the models of the top contestants and their performance during the Chinese diabetes question classification shared task. The participation teams from both industry and academia had achieved commendable results in this classification task. The efforts and outcomes had significantly contributed to the advancement of automatic Chinese diabetes question answering. In addition, an analysis of the methodologies employed by the top-performing teams was conducted. Notably, the top two teams utilized large models for training, further highlighting the immense potential of large models in classification tasks.

Acknowledgments. The work is supported by grants from National Natural Science Foundation of China (62372189), Natural Science Foundation of Guangdong Province (2021A1515220137), the Research Grants Council of the Hong Kong Special Administrative Region, China (UGC/FDS16/E09/22), the Key Research Laboratory Construction Project of National Administration of Traditional Chinese Medicine ([2012]27), and the Project of Traditional Chinese Medicine Bureau of Guangdong Province (20215004).

References

1. Hao, T., Li, X., He, Y., Wang, F.L., Qu, Y.: Recent progress in leveraging deep learning methods for question answering. Neural Comput. Appl. **34**(4), 2765–2783 (2022)
2. Hao, T., Xie, W., Wu, Q., Weng, H., Qu, Y.: Leveraging question target word features through semantic relation expansion for answer type classification. Knowl.-Based Syst. **133**, 43–52 (2017)
3. Liu, Y., Hao, T., Liu, H., Mu, Y., Weng, H., Wang, F.L.: OdeBERT: one-stage deep supervised early-exiting BERT for fast inference in user intent classification. ACM Trans. on Asian Low-Resour. Lang. Inf. Process. **22**(5), 1–18 (2023)
4. Xie, W., Ding, R., Yan, J., et al.: A mobile-based question-answering and early warning system for assisting diabetes management. Wirel. Commun. Mob. Comput. **2018**, 1–14 (2018)
5. Qian, X., Xie, W., Long, S., Lan, M., Mu, Y., Hao, T.: The construction of question taxonomy and an annotated Chinese corpus for diabetes question classification. In: Proceedings of The Chinese National Conference on Computational Linguistics, pp.395–405 (2022)
6. Hochreiter, S., Schmidhuber, J.: Long short-term memory. Neural Comput. **9**(8), 1735–1780 (1997)
7. Kim, Y.: Convolutional neural networks for sentence classification. In: Proceedings of EMNLP, pp. 1746–1751 (2014)
8. Mihalcea, R., Tarau, P.: Textrank: bringing order into text. In: Proceedings of EMNLP, pp. 404–411 (2004)
9. Vaswani, A., Shazeer, N., Parmar, N., et al.: Attention is all you need. In: Advances in neural information processing systems, vol. 30 (2017)
10. Munkhdalai, T., Yu, H.: Neural Semantic Encoders the Conference. Association for Computational Linguistics. Meeting, vol. 1, p. 397. NIH Public Access (2017)
11. Ely, J.W., Osheroff, J.A., Gorman, P.N., et al.: A taxonomy of generic clinical questions: classification study. BMJ **321**(7258), 429–432 (2000)
12. O'Halloran, J., Miller, G.C., Britt, H.: Defining chronic conditions for primary care with ICPC-2. Fam. Pract. **21**(4), 381–386 (2004)
13. McRoy, S., Jones, S., Kurmally, A.: Toward automated classification of consumers' cancer-related questions with a new taxonomy of expected answer types. Health Inform. J. **22**(3), 523–535 (2016)
14. Roberts, K., Masterton, K., Fiszman, M., et al.: Annotating question types for consumer health questions. In: Proceedings of The LREC Workshop on Building and Evaluating Resources for Health and Biomedical Text Processing, pp. 1–8 (2014)
15. Wang, T.H., Zhou, X.F., Ni, Y., et al.: Health information needs regarding diabetes mellitus in China: an internet-based analysis. BMC Public Health **20**(2020), 1–9 (2020)
16. Guo, X., Liang, L., Liu, Y., et al.: The construction of a diabetes-oriented frequently asked question corpus for automated question-answering services. In: Proceedings of the Conference on Artificial Intelligence and Healthcare, pp. 60–66 (2020)
17. McHugh, M.L.: Interrater Reliability: The Kappa Statistic. Biochem. Med. **22**(3), 276–282 (2012)
18. Elliott, A.C., Woodward, W.A.: Statistical Analysis Quick Reference Guidebook: With SPSS Examples. SAGE (2007)
19. Liu, P.F., Qiu, X.P., Huang, X.J.: Recurrent neural network for text classification with multitask learning. In: Proceedings of the Twenty-Fifth International Joint Conference on Artificial Intelligence, pp. 2873–2879 (2016)
20. Devlin, J., Chang, M.W., Lee, K., Toutanova, K.: BERT: pre-training of deep bidirectional transformers for language understanding. In: Proceedings of the Conference of the North American Chapter of the Association for Computational Linguistics, pp. 4171–4186 (2019)

Chinese Diabetes Question Classification Using Large Language Models and Transfer Learning

Chengze Ge[1,2(✉)], Hongshun Ling[1], Fuliang Quan[1], and Jianping Zeng[2]

[1] Huimei Technology, Hangzhou, China
{gechengze,linghongshun,quanfuliang}@huimei.com
[2] School of Computer Science, Fudan University, Shanghai, China
zjp@fudan.edu.cn

Abstract. Type 2 diabetes has evolved into a significant global public health challenge. Diabetes question-answering services are playing an increasingly important role in providing daily health services for patients and high-risk populations. As one of the evaluation track for CHIP 2023, participants are required to classify diabetes-related questions. We have introduced an approach that utilizes generative open-source large language models to accomplish this task. Initially, we designed a prompt construction method that transforms question-label pairs into a conversational text. Subsequently, we fine-tuned the large language model using LoRA method. Furthermore, to enhance the capability in the medical domain, we employed another open-source dataset for initial fine-tuning of the model, followed by transfer learning to fine-tune the Chinese diabetes questions dataset. Experimental results demonstrate the superiority of our approach, ultimately achieving a score of 92.10 on the test data.

Keywords: Diabetes questions classification · LLM · LoRA Fine-Tuning · Transfer Learning

1 Introduction

With the rapid growth of the internet, the increasing demand for diabetes-specific information among the vast population of type 2 diabetes patients and high-risk individuals has become increasingly prominent. Diabetes, as a typical chronic disease, has evolved into a significant global public health challenge. Diabetes automatic question-answering services are playing an increasingly vital role in delivering daily health services to patients and high-risk individuals. The Chinese Diabetes Question Classification Evaluation Task[1] aims to automatically classify questions related to diabetes that patients pose. This task is expected to enhance the performance of search results and drive the development of diabetes automatic question-answering services. The evaluation dataset consists of

---

[1] http://cips-chip.org.cn/2023/eval6.

H. Xu et al. (Eds.): CHIP 2023, CCIS 2080, pp. 205–213, 2024.
https://doi.org/10.1007/978-981-97-1717-0_19

Chinese diabetes questions categorized into a total of six classes, including *diagnosis, treatment, common knowledge, healthy lifestyle, epidemiology,* and *others.* We need to predict the classification of diabetes questions in the test set.

In recent years, with the rapid advancement of Pre-trained Language Models (PLMs) [11,22], the approach of utilizing them for text classification tasks has become increasingly prevalent. Taking BERT [2] as an example, a common practice involves connecting the embedding of the special token [CLS] from a sentence to a fully connected layer to accomplish the classification task. On the other hand, with the emergence of generative large language models, various types of tasks, such as text classification [16] and named entity recognition [20], can be reframed as text generation tasks, often yielding performance on par with or surpassing that of traditional models.

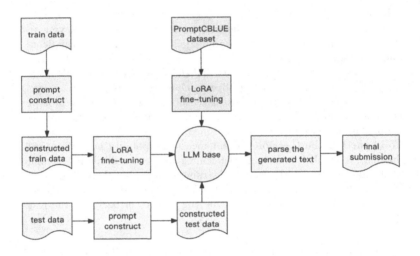

Fig. 1. Overall workflow of our approach. Initially, we fine-tune the open-source large language model using an external dataset, PromptCBLUE [25]. Based on the fine-tuned checkpoint, we further fine-tune the model on the current task dataset using transfer learning. We employ the same prompt construction method for both the training and testing sets, transforming the text classification task into a text generation task. Finally, we map the generated text back to the corresponding label numbers.

To this end, we propose a solution for the evaluation task using a generative large language models (LLM). Furthermore, in order to enhance the capabilities of open-source LLMs in the medical knowledge domain, we leverage additional medical datasets through transfer learning to accomplish this task. In summary, as illustrated in Fig. 1, our approach consists of two parts: **(1) Large Language Model**: To leveraging the characteristics of LLMs, we innovatively transform the text classification problem into a text generation task by designing appropriate prompts and providing a list of candidate categories. This approach aims to minimize the generation of results outside the six specified categories. **(2) Transfer**

Learning: For open-source LLMs, their knowledge in the medical domain might not be as robust. Therefore, we consider employing a transfer learning approach. We introduce an external dataset, PromptCBLUE [25], for fine-tuning on the open-source LLM. Based on the obtained checkpoint, we further fine-tune the data constructed for the current evaluation.

The main contributions of this article are as follows:

- We design an innovative workflow to tackle the task of diabetes question classification.
- The competition results demonstrate the effectiveness of our approach, ultimately achieving a score of 92.10, securing the first place.

2   Related Work

Text classification is a fundamental natural language processing (NLP) task that involves assigning predefined categories or labels to textual documents. Over the years, text classification has gained significant attention and has found applications in various domains, including information retrieval, spam email detection, sentiment analysis, and topic categorization. Many text classification methods have been proposed, ranging from traditional machine learning algorithms such as Naive Bayes [14], Support Vector Machines [5] (SVM), Convolutional Neural Networks [4] (CNNs) and Recurrent Neural Networks [10] (RNNs). However, with the development of pre-trained language models, the paradigm of text classification has gradually converged. Fine-tuning pre-trained models such as BERT [2], RoBERTa [9], ERNIE [17], and others on various classification datasets has become the predominant approach.

In terms of the architecture of the Transformer [19], the BERT [2] model belongs to the encoder, while the GPT [1,12,13] series belongs to the decoder and is primarily used for text generation tasks. In the past few years, there has been rapid development in LLMs. LLMs generally refer to those with parameters numbering over tens of billions. Different research institutions have also contributed many open-source LLMs, such as ChatGLM [3,23], LLaMA [18], Baichuan [21], Bloom [15], and others. Unlike traditional fine-tuning methods, one common approach for LLM fine-tuning is efficient parameter tuning, with the currently most popular methods being LoRA [6] and P-tuning [7,8]. Through the prompt engineering, different NLP tasks such as text classification, named entity recognition, and relation extraction can be transformed into text generation tasks. Sun [16] proposed a text classification method based on large language models in their work, employing a step-by-step reasoning strategy.

3   Methodology

3.1   Prompt Construction

As shown in Table 1, the data provided by the organizers is in tabular format and consists of two columns. The first column contains questions, while the second

Table 1. Original Training Data

Question	Label
空腹78血糖算糖尿病吗? Is a fasting blood sugar level of 78 considered diabetes?	0
减肥后糖尿病会好吗 Will diabetes improve after losing weight?	3

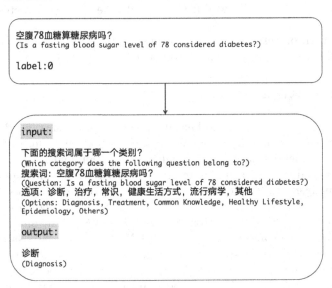

Fig. 2. Prompt Construction Process

column contains category labels ranging from 0 to 5, corresponding to *diagnosis, treatment, common knowledge, healthy lifestyle, epidemiology,* and *others* respectively.

In Fig. 2, we have devised a prompt construction method to transform the raw data into a question-and-answer format. Specifically, the input is divided into three parts. The first part consists of the task description ***Which category does the following question belong to?***, which instructs the model on what task to perform. The second part presents specific search queries. The third part provides candidate options, encompassing all label categories, in order to constrain the generated output of our model within these options as much as possible. The output part is relatively straightforward, as it directly provides the Chinese text for the category.

3.2   Supervised Fine-Tuning

SFT (Supervised Fine-Tuning) involves refining the parameters of a source pretrained model on labeled data to create a new model. Specifically, SFT consists of the following three steps:

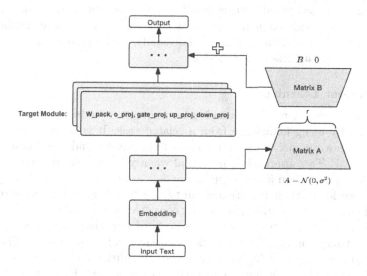

Fig. 3. LoRA Fine-tuning Process

- **Pre-training:** Initially, a model is trained on a large-scale dataset, typically using self-supervised or unsupervised learning algorithms for pre-training. There are currently numerous large language models, both open-source and proprietary, such as GPT-3 [1], ChatGPT-130B [23], LLaMA [18], and others. These models can be categorized based on their architecture into Causal Decoder, Prefix Decoder, and Encoder-Decoder. Furthermore, they differ in their usage of position encoding, activation functions, and normalization methods [24]. In this experiment, we selected **Baichuan2-13B** as the base model. The reason for this choice is that the model size is well-suited for our hardware, and through experimental comparisons, it has demonstrated favorable performance in the current task.
- **Fine-tuning:** To address the challenge of fine-tuning models with an excessive number of parameters while maintaining effectiveness, several parameter-efficient fine-tuning methods have surfaced, with mainstream approaches including LoRA [6] and P-tuning [7,8]. In this task, we chose the LoRA efficient parameter fine-tuning method. The reason for this choice is that, through comparisons, we found that LoRA outperforms P-Tuning in this task. Specifically, as illustrated in Fig. 3, we selected the target modules of the base model. For these modules, we introduced a side-branch, set a LoRA rank, and performed dimensionality reduction followed by dimensionality expansion. We initialized matrix A with a random Gaussian distribution and matrix B with a zero matrix, ensuring that at the beginning of training, this side-branch matrix remains a zero matrix. Through experimental trials, We set the target modules as W_pack, o_proj, gate_proj, up_proj, and down_proj, with a LoRA rank set to 8.

- **Evaluation:** Before submitting results, we assessed the performance using a validation set and conducted activities such as hyperparameter tuning, bad case analysis, and data cleaning. Additionally, we employed cross-validation to enhance robustness of our model.

3.3 Transfer Learning

Transfer learning is a machine learning technique that improves performance of a new task by using knowledge from a related task. It is widely used in deep learning, where a model is first trained on a large dataset and then fine-tuned for a specific task. This approach is beneficial when you have limited data for your task. Since open-source large language models are typically trained on general domain knowledge, their performance in the medical field is not very strong. In this evaluation task, the training dataset consisted of only 6,000 samples, which is relatively small in comparison to the scale of large language models. Thus, direct fine-tuning on this limited data can easily lead to overfitting. Therefore, we employed transfer learning to enhance the capabilities of the open-source large models in the medical domain. We utilized another dataset, PromptCBLUE-v2[2], to first perform SFT on Baichuan2-13B. Based on the obtained checkpoint, we further fine-tuned the model on a diabetes classification dataset. We observed that, compared to direct fine-tuning from the open-source Baichuan2-13B model, this transfer learning approach resulted in superior model performance.

The PromptCBLUE-v2 evaluation benchmark is an advanced version of the CBLUE benchmark, where all 18 different NLP tasks in various medical scenarios have been transformed into prompt-based language generation tasks. This development establishes the first Chinese medical scene benchmark for large language models. The way we construct prompts for this task is similar to PromptCBLUE, allowing for effective utilization of transfer learning and making the most of the high-quality medical domain knowledge representations acquired from PromptCBLUE.

4 Experiments

4.1 Evaluation Metrics

As shown in Eq. 1, Accuracy (Acc) is a widely used evaluation metric in machine learning and classification tasks. It measures the proportion of correctly classified instances or samples in a dataset.

$$\text{Acc} = \frac{\text{Number of Correctly Classified Samples}}{\text{Total Number of Samples}} \times 100\% \tag{1}$$

4.2 Experimental Setup

Our experimental environment was CentOS 7, with a single A800 GPU running CUDA version 12.0. The hyper parameters were configured as presented in Table 2.

---

[2] https://tianchi.aliyun.com/competition/entrance/532132.

Table 2. Hyper Parameters

Hyper Parameters	Value
LoRA target module	W_pack,o_proj,gate_proj,up_proj,down_proj
LoRA rank	8
learning rate	5e−5
lr scheduler	cosine
batch size	8
gradient accumulation steps	4
epoch	10

4.3 Experimental Results

Our model achieved a score of 92.10 on the final test data. In addition, we conducted relevant ablation experiments, as shown in Table 3. Without the use of SFT on the PromptCBLUE data for transfer learning, the score was 90.80. This improvement was due to the successful acquisition of medical domain knowledge through transfer learning. The experimental results regarding the hyperparameter *LoRA rank* are presented in Table 3. We ultimately found that setting *LoRA rank* to 8 produced the best model performance. We attribute this to the relatively short context length of the task data, as setting *LoRA rank* too high could lead to overfitting. Therefore, 8 is a more suitable value.

Furthermore, we conducted experiments with conventional text classification models. We fine-tuned three pretrained models, namely BERT-base-chinese, RoBERTa-chinese, and ERNIE, as shown in Table 3, and achieved scores of 89.90, 90.80, and 90.60, respectively. It can be concluded that while employing larger models ultimately leads to higher scores, the advantage is not substantial.

Table 3. Experimental Results

	Value	Acc
Transfer Learning	No	90.80
	Yes	**92.10**
LoRA rank	16	91.40
	32	91.20
	8	**92.10**
Model	BERT-base-chinese	89.90
	RoBERTa-chinese	90.80
	ERNIE	90.60
	Baichuan2-13B	**92.10**

5   Conclusion

In summary, to address the task of Chinese diabetes question classification, we have proposed a method that utilizes large language models. Firstly, in order to employ generative large language models for classification tasks, we devised a prompt construction method that transforms question-label pairs into conversational data with prompts. Subsequently, to fine-tune the model using the constructed data, we adopted the LoRA fine-tuning approach. Additionally, to enhance the performance in the medical domain of the open-source large language model, we initially fine-tuned it on a more extensive medical domain dataset, PromptCBLUE, and then fine-tuned it further for Chinese diabetes questions using transfer learning. Experimental results demonstrate the effectiveness of our approach.

Limitation. Despite the promising results and contributions of our study, it is essential to acknowledge several limitations. First, compared to the huge number of parameters in large language models, it requires more hardware and resources, but does not have an overwhelming advantage over traditional classification models. Second, the prompt construction method is relatively simple, and more construction methods can be tried in the future to observe whether the effect can be improved.

References

1. Brown, T., et al.: Language models are few-shot learners. Adv. Neural. Inf. Process. Syst. **33**, 1877–1901 (2020)
2. Devlin, J., Chang, M., Lee, K., Toutanova, K.: BERT: pre-training of deep bidirectional transformers for language understanding. In: Burstein, J., Doran, C., Solorio, T. (eds.) Proceedings of the 2019 Conference of the North American Chapter of the Association for Computational Linguistics: Human Language Technologies, NAACL-HLT 2019, Minneapolis, MN, USA, June 2–7, 2019, Volume 1 (Long and Short Papers). pp. 4171–4186. Association for Computational Linguistics (2019). https://doi.org/10.18653/V1/N19-1423
3. Du, Z., et al.: GLM: General language model pretraining with autoregressive blank infilling. In: Proceedings of the 60th Annual Meeting of the Association for Computational Linguistics (Volume 1: Long Papers), pp. 320–335. Association for Computational Linguistics, Dublin, Ireland (2022). https://doi.org/10.18653/v1/2022.acl-long.26, https://aclanthology.org/2022.acl-long.26
4. Gu, J., et al.: Recent advances in convolutional neural networks. Pattern Recogn. **77**, 354–377 (2018)
5. Hearst, M.A., Dumais, S.T., Osuna, E., Platt, J., Scholkopf, B.: Support vector machines. IEEE Intell. Syst. Appl. **13**, 18–28 (1998)
6. Hu, E.J., et al.: Lora: low-rank adaptation of large language models. In: The Tenth International Conference on Learning Representations, ICLR 2022, Virtual Event, April 25–29, 2022. OpenReview.net (2022). https://openreview.net/forum?id=nZeVKeeFYf9

7. Liu, X., et al.: P-tuning: prompt tuning can be comparable to fine-tuning across scales and tasks. In: Proceedings of the 60th Annual Meeting of the Association for Computational Linguistics (Volume 2: Short Papers), ACL 2022, Dublin, Ireland, May 22–27, 2022, pp. 61–68. Association for Computational Linguistics (2022). https://doi.org/10.18653/v1/2022.acl-short.8

8. Liu, X., et al.: GPT understands, too. CoRR abs/2103.10385 (2021). https://arxiv.org/abs/2103.10385

9. Liu, Y., et al.: Roberta: a robustly optimized bert pretraining approach. arXiv preprint arXiv:1907.11692 (2019)

10. Medsker, L.R., Jain, L.: Recurrent neural networks. Des. Appl. 5(64–67), 2 (2001)

11. Min, B., et al.: Recent advances in natural language processing via large pre-trained language models: a survey. ACM Comput. Surv. 56(2), 1–40 (2023)

12. Radford, A., Narasimhan, K., Salimans, T., Sutskever, I., et al.: Improving language understanding by generative pre-training (2018)

13. Radford, A., Wu, J., Child, R., Luan, D., Amodei, D., Sutskever, I., et al.: Language models are unsupervised multitask learners. OpenAI blog 1(8), 9 (2019)

14. Rish, I., et al.: An empirical study of the naive bayes classifier. In: IJCAI 2001 Workshop on Empirical Methods in Artificial Intelligence, vol. 3, pp. 41–46 (2001)

15. Scao, T.L., et al.: Bloom: a 176b-parameter open-access multilingual language model (2023)

16. Sun, X., et al.: Text classification via large language models. arXiv preprint arXiv:2305.08377 (2023)

17. Sun, Y., et al.: Ernie 2.0: a continual pre-training framework for language understanding. In: Proceedings of the AAAI Conference on Artificial Intelligence. vol. 34, pp. 8968–8975 (2020)

18. Touvron, H., et al.: Llama: open and efficient foundation language models (2023)

19. Vaswani, A., et al.: Attention is all you need. In: Advances in Neural Information Processing Systems, vol. 30 (2017)

20. Wang, S., et al.: Gpt-ner: named entity recognition via large language models. arXiv preprint arXiv:2304.10428 (2023)

21. Yang, A., et al.: Baichuan 2: open large-scale language models. arXiv preprint arXiv:2309.10305 (2023)

22. Yang, S., Feng, D., Qiao, L., Kan, Z., Li, D.: Exploring pre-trained language models for event extraction and generation. In: Proceedings of the 57th Annual Meeting of the Association for Computational Linguistics, pp. 5284–5294 (2019)

23. Zeng, A., et al.: GLM-130b: an open bilingual pre-trained model. In: The Eleventh International Conference on Learning Representations (ICLR) (2023)

24. Zhao, W.X., et al.: A survey of large language models (2023)

25. Zhu, W., Wang, X., Zheng, H., Chen, M., Tang, B.: Promptcblue: a Chinese prompt tuning benchmark for the medical domain (2023)

A Model Ensemble Approach with LLM for Chinese Text Classification

Chengyan Wu[1], Wenlong Fang[1], Feipeng Dai[1(✉)], and Hailong Yin[2]

[1] School of Electronics and Information Engineering,
South China Normal University, Foshan 528225, China
`chengyan.wu@m.scnu.edu.cn, daifeipeng@126.com`
[2] Institute for Brain Research and Rehabilitation,
South China Normal University, Guangzhou 510631, China

Abstract. Automatic medical text categorization can assist doctors in efficiently managing patient information. By categorizing textual information such as patients' descriptions of symptoms, doctors can easily find key information, accelerate the diagnostic process, provide superior medical advice, and successfully promote smart diagnosis and medical automated QA services. In this paper, an approach to medical text categorization is presented in the open-share task of the 9th China Conference on Health Information Processing (CHIP 2023), where complex textual relations are the two main challenges of this task. A model integration approach is proposed for this task, which can effectively solve medical text categorization through the complementary relationship of three different submodels. In addition, the solution provides external tools for targeted data enhancement for difficult samples that are hard to classify to reduce misclassification. Final results are obtained by the models through a voting mechanism. Experimental results show that the proposed method can achieve 92% accuracy and also prove the effectiveness of the model.

Keywords: Medical text categorization · Large language models · Adversarial training · Data augmentation · External tools for large language models

1 Introduction

With the rapid development of medical automated question-and-answer services, automatically analyzing medical texts, archiving patient records, automated diagnosis, and automatic classification have significantly progressed. This advancement facilitates fast and accurate diagnoses for various diseases. In particular, text classification plays a crucial role in clinical record organization and retrieval, supporting queue identification and clinical decision-making [1,2]. Existing research on clinical text classification often involves feature engineering

---

C. Wu and W. Fang—These authors contributed equally to this work.

© The Author(s), under exclusive license to Springer Nature Singapore Pte Ltd. 2024
H. Xu et al. (Eds.): CHIP 2023, CCIS 2080, pp. 214–230, 2024.
https://doi.org/10.1007/978-981-97-1717-0_20

using different forms of rules or knowledge sources [3–7]. However, most studies struggle to automatically learn effective features, while recent advancements in deep learning methods [8] have demonstrated powerful capabilities in automatic text classification. Automatic text classification involves prejudging and categorizing patient inquiry questions, aiding in the establishment of highly effective doctor- patient communication channels within limited medical time. Consequently, this classification helps doctors quickly understand the main issues of patients, facilitating the formulation of medical decisions. Simultaneously, automatic text classification enables doctors to conduct inquiries systematically, thus efficiently acquiring key information.

The 9th China Health Information Processing Conference (CHIP 2023) is an annual event organized by the Medical Health and Bioinformatics Processing Professional Committee of the China Information Processing Society (CIPS), with the theme of "Exploring the Mysteries of Life, Improving Health Quality, and Enhancing Medical Standards with Information Processing Technology." The conference includes six tasks, with Task 6 focusing on Chinese diabetes question classification. The categories for this task encompass diagnosis, treatment, common knowledge, healthy lifestyle, epidemiology, and others. Text classification is a traditional supervised learning task where algorithms are trained to automatically categorize text into different classes. In the medical field, which involves numerous specialized terms and domain knowledge, models with strong semantic understanding capabilities are often required to handle these complex semantic scenarios effectively. Text classification models with a small number of parameters may yield unsatisfactory results. Therefore, in medical text classification [9], introducing language models with large parameter sizes and strong semantic understanding capabilities is crucial. Additionally, in the medical domain, the labeled data used for training may exhibit local differences with inconsistent labels due to the diverse forms of medical inquiry data. This diversity poses challenges in classifying difficult samples in medical inquiry text classification, necessitating effective data augmentation strategies for model training. Moreover, traditional single-model text classification often lacks interpretability and may lead to misclassifications, especially in the stringent medical field. The performance of a single model may decline rapidly due to different text distributions in the training data. Therefore, a comprehensive evaluation of multiple models is often preferable. Furthermore, regarding the finetuning of large models, complete finetuning yields superior results but consumes additional resources and time.

This paper investigates model integration and voting mechanism methods for the diabetes dataset provided by the organizer to solve the above problems. This paper is based on the framework of large-model external tools to address the uneven distribution of some samples and the difficulty of classification. These tools can be targeted to extract difficult samples that are difficult to classify and augment (that is, to solve the problem of uneven samples and deal with the misclassified samples). In terms of model finetuning, a variety of three frameworks, including LoRA, QLoRA, and FGM, are used to finetune the three models, which solves the problem of excessive cost and time due to full-volume finetuning. These frameworks can also be highly efficient. Simultaneously, adversarial training with perturbation is introduced to the small model, which can successfully identify the subtle differences between difficult samples and effectively improve the classification accuracy and the robustness of the model. When the model finally decides, the strategy of majority voting is applied to solve the instability of single-model direct classification. Overall, this paper adopts Qwen-7b-Chat, ChatGLM2-6b, and MacBERT as the base models and utilizes the external tools Claude2 and ChatGPT to assist in data enhancement. The paper also utilizes QLoRA and LoRA frameworks to finetune the command of SFT for the large model, merge the finetuned parameters, and then perform batch inference. FGM adversarial training is used to train the small model. The base large model performs the good multiple choice task, and the small model performs the traditional text label classification to complete the classification task together, finally achieving an accuracy of 0.92 on the test set.

The main contributions of this work are as follows:

- The model integration method is formulated for text classification. A method of combining small models with large language-pretrained models is proposed in this paper to solve the misclassification of single model classifications through the respective advantages of large and small models.
- The method of calling external tools to perform data enhancement for difficult samples in an uneven sample distribution is proposed to solve the misclassification problem of difficult samples.
- A voting mechanism is applied to the model outputs. The results indicate that when incorporating a voting mechanism on top of data augmentation, in terms of accuracy for the test and validation datasets, the approach with the voting mechanism outperforms the method of solely conducting data augmentation by 0.8%–1.1%.

2   Related Work

2.1   Text Classification

Medical text categorization has attracted considerable attention in the field of NLP, and researchers have mainly utilized medical text datasets for tasks such as disease classification and diagnosis. The main approaches include feature extraction, machine learning, and deep learning methods. Traditional text classification models prefer using feature engineering methods, where text is first represented as vectors and then machine learning algorithms are used to implement the classification process. CNN and RNN are some of the most representative deep learning models. CNN learn to recognize patterns across space [10], increasing their effectiveness in tasks such as detecting localized and position-invariant patterns. Kalchbrenner et al. [11] first proposed a CNN-based text categorization model called Dynamic CNN (DCNN). DCNN induces feature maps on sentences to capture word relationships of different sizes. Kim [12] proposed a model that uses only one layer of convolution on word vectors obtained from unsupervised neurolinguistic models (e.g., word2vec). Therefore, several researchers have investigated improvements to CNN-based models. RNN [13] are trained to recognize patterns across time, increasing their suitability for tasks such as understanding remote semantics. Tai et al. [14] proposed to generalize the LSTM [15] to a tree-structured network type called Tree-LSTM. The Tree-LSTM is highly effective for sentiment classification and correlation, with better effectiveness than previous systems. Liu et al. [16] proposed three different information sharing mechanisms. The voting mechanism is an integrated learning approach in medical text categorization; in [9], Valdovinos used a multiple-classifier system with majority voting. Since 2018, pretraining and finetuning have become one of the most commonly used methods in NLP tasks due to BERT, which was proposed by Devlin et al. [17]. These methods have also displayed significant benefits in downstream classification tasks.

2.2 Adversarial Training

With the development of deep learning, adversarial training has received considerable attention. In recent years, with the increasing difficulty of generating effective adversarial samples in natural language tasks and other related problems, adversarial training has been introduced in the field of natural language processing (NLP), such as domain adaptation [18], cross-linguistic transfer learning [19], and multitask learning [20], where adversarial training enhances the robustness of the model through adversarial attacks and defenses. Szegedy et al. [21] first introduced the concept of adversarial samples and formed adversarial samples by adding some subtle disturbances to the dataset. Goodfellow et al. [22] first introduced the concept of adversarial training and devised a fast gradient symbol method (FGSM) to compute disturbances in the input samples. Miyato et al. [23] made some modifications to the part of FGSM to compute the interference, normalized it according to a specific gradient, suggested adding interference to the word vector layer, and performed a semi-supervised text classification task to verify its effectiveness. In addition, an approach based on local adversarial training by Li Jing et al. [24] not only mitigates the named entity recognition problem caused by boundary sample confusion but also reduces the redundancy of adversarial samples due to the increased computation in traditional adversarial training. Yasunaga et al. [25] used adversarial training in a POS task, which not only improves the overall labeling accuracy but also enhances the robustness of the model. Zhou et al. [26] added interference to the word embedding layer, which improved the generalization of named entity recognition models with few resources.

2.3 Fine-Tuning of Large Language Models

Large model fine-tuning refers to further training based on a pre-trained large neural network model by using a task-specific small-scale dataset in order to adapt the model to the specific characteristics of the task. This fine-tuning strategy is widely used in deep learning, especially in the field of natural language processing (NLP). One work proposes regularization methods to improve generalization and calibration during fine-tuning of language models. For example, Wang et al. [27] explored the combination of KL and L2 regularization on extracted features to preserve the calibration of pre-trained masked language models (MLMs). Li et al. [28] and Aghajanyan et al. [29] have showed that learned over-parametrized models are actually present in low intrinsic dimensions, and that LoRA allows for a rank decomposition through optimization of the dense layer changes during the adaptation of the matrix to indirectly train some of the dense layers in the neural network while keeping the pre-trained weight frozen, which makes LoRA both storage and computationally efficient.

2.4   Data Augmentation

Most machine and deep learning-based models currently require a large expansion of the corpus. Previous work has proposed several techniques for data augmentation in NLP. Yu et al. generated new data by translating sentences into French and back into English [30]. Xie et al.'s work used data Pilots as a predictive language model for smoothing [31] and synonym substitution [32]. Wei et al. proposed a simple set of generalized data augmentation techniques for NLP [33] called EDA, which is the first work to fully explore data-enabled text editing techniques. These methods aim to address the problem of relatively limited amount of data and improve the performance and generalization of deep learning models through data augmentation.

2.5   Prompt Engineering

Prompt engineering provides humans with a natural and intuitive interface for interacting with and using generic models such as LLM. The prompts proposed by Timo et al. have been widely used as a generalized method for NLP tasks due to their flexibility [34]. However, LLMs require proper cue engineering, either manually [35] or automatically [36], because models do not understand cues as well as humans. Liu et al. proposed several successful fast-tuning methods using gradient-based methods for optimization over continuous spaces [37]. However, as computing gradients becomes highly expensive, moving access to models to APIs that may not provide gradient access becomes increasingly difficult as the scale becomes gradually impractical.

3   Proposed Methodology

3.1   Model Structure

This section describes the ensemble model designed for the diabetes question classification problem. The overall structure of the model is shown in Fig. 1 and mainly comprises three major components: the model ensemble, data augmentation, and a voting mechanism. In the model ensemble component, Qwen-7b-Chat,

ChatGLM2-6b, and MacBERT are utilized as base models. The QLoRA and LoRA frameworks are employed for supervised fine-tuning instructions on large models, and batch inference is conducted after merging the fine-tuned parameters. Adversarial training using the fast gradient method (FGM) is applied to train small models. The base large models specialize in multiple-choice tasks, while the small models handle traditional text label classification, collectively contributing to the overall task. In the data augmentation component, a filter is used to identify misclassified samples after obtaining model output results.

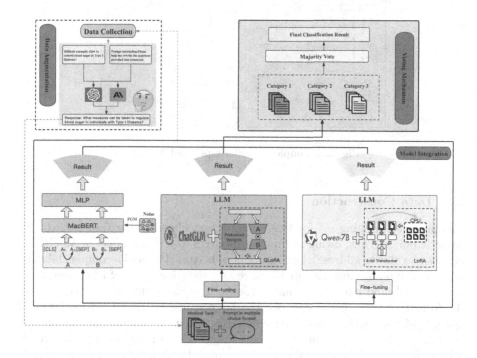

Fig. 1. The architecture and pipeline of the proposed integrated model.

External tools are then employed to perform paraphrasing on these samples, and the augmented samples are added to the original training dataset. For the voting mechanism, each of the three base models produces classification results. The classification results are aggregated through a majority voting approach, and the majority class is determined as the final output, resulting in the ultimate classification outcome.

3.2   Problem Description

Formally, given an input sentence $s = \{w_1, \ldots, w_L\}$, w_i denotes the i-th token of the sequence. The diabetes text categorization task aims to classify the input sentences into predefined categories, i.e., Diagnosis, Treatment, Common Knowledge, healthy lifestyle, Epidemiology, and Other, which correspond to the numerical labels 0, 1, 2, 3, 4, and 5, respectively. The final output needs to be classified according to $s = \{w_1, \ldots, w_L\}$, and the output needs to be labeled according to $s = \{w_1, \ldots, w_L\}$. The output should be in the format $s = \{\text{sentence, label}\}$. The input and output of the model are shown in Fig. 2 below:

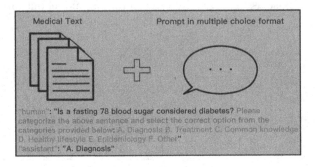

Fig. 2. Example of model input and output.

3.3   Data Construction

The provided training set for this diabetic text classification task is text plus numeric labels. Thus, owing to limited resources, the small model of MacBERT may not be able to address a large amount of textual data and a complex labeling system. The use of numeric labels can reduce the complexity of labels and facilitate a quick and efficient training process. Therefore, this experiment retains the format of the original data for the large models (ChatGLM2-6B [38] and Qwen-7B-Chat), which usually have powerful semantic understanding. Converting numeric labels into multiple-choice questions with content can effectively utilize the semantic understanding of the model and facilitate its comprehensive understanding of the meaning of the text. Therefore, the numeric labels are mapped into a multiple-choice format during the experiments. This format may introduce some benefits over the numeric format when using the large models for text categorization tasks. First, the multiple-choice format is close to the human way of expression and comprehension because people are generally more likely to understand alphabetic labels than abstract numeric labels. This format facilitates a natural and intuitive observation and interpretation of the results for the user. Simultaneously, the format improves the readability and interpretability of the results, and recognizing the meaning of each category in the results without having to look up the correspondence of the numerical labels is easy for the model.

3.4 Data Augmentation

Quantitative analysis was performed on the basis of the provided samples, revealing significant disparities in quantity among the categories of diagnosis, epidemiology, and others compared to treatment, medical knowledge, and a healthy lifestyle. A visual experiment with sentence embeddings revealed that some samples with different labels were clustered together. In the experiment, misclassified samples from the validation set were filtered out. Using a text similarity calculation, similar samples were identified in the training set. An external tool was employed to perform paraphrasing on these challenging samples; however, the meaning of the sentences should remain unchanged. Synonymous sentences were generated through word replacement, random insertion and deletion of phrases, shuffling word order, and structural transformations in syntax. These newly generated synonymous sentences were appropriately added to the original training dataset.

3.5 Model Integration

This paper uses Qwen-7b-Chat, ChatGLM2-6b, and MacBERT as base models for the diabetic text classification task. Different finetuning training methods were used for each of the three different models.

MacBERT. MacBERT is a Chinese pretraining model released by HIT and KDDI, which mainly modifies the MLM task of BERT. Compared with the previous masking method, MacBERT uses N-gram masking when performing [MASK] on the particle words, in which the probability of 1-gram and 4-gram masking is 40%, 30%, 20%, and 10%. This whole-gram masking allows the model to effectively learn the word boundary information and improve semantic understanding [39]. Meanwhile, the use of words with similar meanings to replace those masked by the (MASK) token alleviates the inconsistency between the pretraining and downstream finetuning tasks. MacBERT exhibits relatively superior expressive power in Chinese and allows for an improved understanding of phrase-level semantics. Thus, MacBERT was chosen as one of the models for the current classification task.

FGM. During the training of MacBERT, considering the presence of certain samples in the dataset with different labels but clustered into the same cluster, this study adopted the FGM [23] adversarial training method. This approach aimed to enhance the robustness and classification accuracy of the model by introducing perturbations into the samples, addressing the challenge of classifying subtle differences in difficult samples. FGM is a simple yet effective technique in adversarial training. This method calculates the gradient of the model on the input to generate adversarial perturbations, which are then added to the original samples to improve the robustness of the deep learning model to minor perturbations. This method also introduces adversarial examples during training, increasing the resilience of the model to adversarial attacks. FGM is a common method used to enhance model security and robustness. The working principle is as follows: first, adversarial examples must be generated. For a given input sample X, model f, and loss function J, the gradient of the input is computed considering the loss function:

$$\nabla_X J(f(X), Y), \tag{1}$$

where Y is the true label of the sample. The gradient calculated above is then added as a perturbation to the original sample:

$$\epsilon \cdot \text{sign}\left(\nabla_X J(f(X), Y)\right). \tag{2}$$

The generated adversarial perturbation is added to the original input sample, where ϵ is the size of the perturbation:

$$X_{\text{adv}} = X + \epsilon \cdot \text{sign}\left(\nabla_X J(f(X), Y)\right). \tag{3}$$

Finally, the adversarial sample X_{adv} is used for training along with the original sample X to improve the robustness of the model to adversarial perturbations.

ChatGLM2-6B. ChatGLM2-6B [38] has been optimized for Chinese question answering and dialogue, undergoing approximately one trillion bilingual token training in Chinese and English. Leveraging techniques such as supervised fine-tuning, human feedback reinforcement learning can help generate responses that align well with human preferences. The design background of GLM overcomes the three-way division in traditional pretrained models by integrating the advantages of autoregressive, autoencoding, and encoder-decoder models. Based on the autoregressive blank infilling method, a novel approach that combines the strengths of the three pre-training models is employed, resulting in impressive performance across various Chinese tasks.

Qwen-7B-Chat. QWen-7B is a pretrained language model based on Transformer and is structured on a similar architecture as LLaMA. Pretraining uses data from over 2.2 trillion publicly available tokens and 2048 context lengths. The training data cover general and specialized domains, focusing on English and Chinese in terms of language. Qwen-7B-Chat [40] is finetuned to match human intent through an alignment mechanism that includes task-oriented data as well as specific security- and service-oriented data. From the perspective of Chinese performance in various tasks with comparable parameter magnitudes, Qwen-7B-Chat outperforms other models in various metrics. Therefore, this paper chooses it as one of the large models.

LoRA. LoRA is adopted in the finetuning framework to minimize the need for continuous finetuning of trainable parameters in large model adaptation [41], offering a streamlined approach while maintaining the integrity of pretrained knowledge. Rather than directly finetuning all parameters, the core concept of LoRA involves optimizing a low-rank matrix that captures the changes in weights during the adaptation process. This strategy allows the introduction of trainable parameters during the adaptation to a new task while maintaining the pretrained weights. In LoRA, the weights of the pretrained model are frozen; thus, they no longer receive gradient updates. Therefore, the foundational knowledge of the model remains largely unchanged, adapting to new tasks by introducing additional trainable parameters. This approach reduces the number of trainable parameters that need finetuning in downstream tasks.

QLoRA. QLoRA introduces double quantization to minimize overhead from additional quantization constants. After the first quantization, constants are re-quantized to lower precision, reducing bit requirements. Utilizing a paged opti-mizer, QLoRA allows moving and reloading the optimizer state to manage GPU memory usage peaks [42]. Double quantization decreases bit usage, reducing storage demands. The paging optimizer efficiently handles memory limitations. Bitwise quantization maintains parameter distribution, ensuring consistency and avoiding significant changes in the overall distribution.

3.6   External Tool Utilization

Utilizing external tools by large models is a common practice in NLP and other related fields [43]. In this classification task, external tools such as ChatGPT and Claude2 were employed for data augmentation to precisely distinguish challeng-ing samples and address the difficulty in their classification. After collecting the challenging samples, appropriate prompts were used to guide the external tools in transforming some queries into synonymous sentences, generating a batch of new data for augmentation purposes. For tasks such as medical inquiries, large models demand external tools to obtain a variety of inquiry statements, which is proven beneficial for effectively categorizing issues for targeted treat-ment. This approach enhances the understanding and analysis of key aspects of patient inquiries, aligning well with the displayed scenarios. Diverse training samples contribute to improving the generalization performance of the model. The model becomes suitably equipped to handle unseen inputs by mimicking the diversity in real-world scenarios, significantly contributing to the accuracy of model classification.

3.7   Voting Mechanism

The voting mechanism is commonly employed in text classification within the field of Natural Language Processing to integrate predictions from multiple mod-els [44]. This approach is useful for combining different text classification models, each potentially focusing on different aspects of the training data. An illustration of the majority voting strategy is provided in the Fig. 3 below:

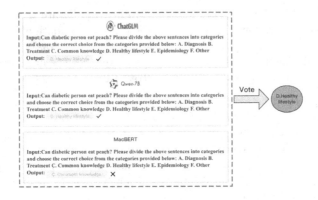

Fig. 3. Voting Mechanism.

These models may utilize different algorithms or feature representations. In the current text classification task, considering that each model has its own strengths and individual model predictions may exhibit instability, a majority voting strategy was adopted. Each voter was given equal voting rights in this task, and the final classification result was determined by the majority of model predictions. In special cases where the results of three voters are inconsistent, the classification result of the model with the highest accuracy on the validation set was chosen as the ultimate output. This approach helps mitigate overfitting of a single model to specific features of the training data, thereby enhancing classification performance.

4   Experiments

4.1   Data Analysis

The dataset is derived from Task 6 of CHIP 2023. The training data comprises 6,000 texts related to diabetes, with annotations for six types of diabetes texts, including Diagnosis, Treatment, Common Knowledge, Healthy Lifestyle, Epidemiology, and Other.

Table 1. Quantitative analysis of raw data.

Type	Diagnosis	Treatment	Common Knowledge	Healthy Lifestyle	Epidemiology	Other
Train	527	1501	1226	1702	599	445

Table 2. Quantitative analysis of data after data augmentation.

Type	Diagnosis	Treatment	Common Knowledge	Healthy Lifestyle	Epidemiology	Other
Train	827	1708	1426	1802	999	1045

First, this paper uses the original dataset for classification. Besides, it uses the data augmentation method to extend the data due to the existence of some samples that are difficult to classify in the original dataset. The statistical information of the dataset before and after data augmentation is respectively shown in Table 1 and Table 2.

4.2 Parameter Settings

In this text classification task, we used three model integrations of MacBERT + ChatGLM2-6B + Qwen-7B-Chat, where, for the large models ChatGLM2-6B and Qwen-7B-Chat, the learning rate is set to 2e−4, the batch size is 12, and epoch is 8. The deep learning framework we used is PyTorch. For the MacBERT model, the learning rate is set to 1e−5, the batch size is 6, and epoch is 8. The parameters of the specific model are shown in Table 3.

Table 3. Experimental parameter settings.

ChatGLM2-6B Qwen-7B-Chat	learning rate	2×10^{-4}
	epoch	8
	batch_size	12
	LoRA_rank	64
	LoRA_alpha	16
	LoRA_dropout	0.05
MacBERT	learning rate	1×10^{-5}
	epoch	8
	batch_size	6

4.3 Evaluation Indicators

This diabetes problem classification task uses accuracy (Acc) to evaluate model performance on the test dataset. The accuracy is described below:

$$\text{Accuracy} = \frac{\text{Number of Correctly Classified Samples}}{\text{Total Number of Samples}} \times 100\% \qquad (4)$$

where Number of Correctly Classified Samples in the numerator represents the instances where the model correctly classified the data points according to their true labels. The Total Number of Samples in the denominator is the sum of correct and incorrect predictions made by the model.

4.4 Results

Table 4 shows the performance comparison between using data augmentation and voting mechanism after integrating the model.

Table 4. Final results of the experiment.

Method	Data	Acc
MacBERT(FGM)+ChatGLM2-6B(QLoRA)+Qwen-7B-Chat(LoRA)+Vote	Val	0.887
	Test	0.899
MacBERT(FGM)+ChatGLM2-6B(QLoRA)+Qwen-7B-Chat(LoRA)+EDA	Val	0.898
	Test	0.909
MacBERT(FGM)+ChatGLM2-6B(QLoRA)+Qwen-7B-Chat(LoRA)+Vote+EDA	Val	**0.906**
	Test	**0.92**

As shown in the table, the model with data augmentation(EDA) is superior in Acc on both datasets compared to that with the voting mechanism. This superiority proves that a large positive ground boost is obtained by performing data augmentation on difficult samples. Specifically, the model with data augmentation achieves 89.8% and 90.9% accuracy on the two datasets. The following observations are also presented. The accuracy of the classification results by the three models with the introduction of the voting mechanism and data augmentation is higher than that of data augmentation and majority voting alone; specifically, the models with the addition of data augmentation and majority voting achieve 90.6% and 92.0% accuracy on the two datasets, respectively. These results are mainly due to the following: 1) Data augmentation can generate additional samples by introducing various text transformations, allowing the model to be exposed to a large diversity of data during training. Such exposure helps the model effectively capture the differences between different inputs and improves the generalization capability. 2) If labeling errors or noises exist in the training data, then data enhancement helps reduce the impact of these noises. The model is more likely to learn real patterns rather than errors in the training data by introducing diversity in the data augmentation process. 3) The advantage of data augmentation lies in the superiority of the model to adapt to diversity by augmenting the training data, thus improving its performance and robustness. In most votes, while robustness can be improved by integrating the results of multiple models, data augmentation may be highly effective when data are limited or noisy. 4) Using a model that combines the two approaches not only helps the model to effectively capture differences between inputs but also synthesizes a bit of each model and reduces misclassification from a single model.

4.5 Ablation Experiments

Eleven sets of experiments are conducted to further assess the effectiveness of each model within the ensemble. Ablation studies are performed individually using the three base models in the validation and test sets. As shown in Table 5, for the small model MacBERT, incorporating FGM adversarial training during the training phase effectively enhances its performance. This finding suggests that introducing perturbation information can alleviate issues related to an uneven sample distribution. Furthermore, for the large models ChatGLM2-

6B and Qwen-7B-Chat, significant improvements in classification accuracy are observed after finetuning the models using the LoRA and QLoRA frameworks. This indicates that fine-tuning pre-trained large models enables them to adapt to specific domain tasks. Examining the finetuning effects under different frameworks, QLoRA framework finetuning on ChatGLM2-6B shows superior performance, possibly due to the introduction of additional parameters with the inserted adapter layer in QLoRA. LoRA framework finetuning on Qwen-7B-Chat also exhibits superior results. Additionally, data augmentation is individually applied to each of the three base models, resulting in varying degrees of improvement in Acc scores. This finding suggests that the augmentation approach effectively expands the quantity of difficult samples.

Table 5. Results of comparison of different models and methods.

Method	Data	Acc
MacBERT	Val	0.87
	Test	0.89
MacBERT+FGM	Val	0.876
	Test	0.897
MacBERT+EDA	Val	0.877
	Test	0.899
ChaGLM2-6B	Val	0.874
	Test	0.89
ChaGLM2-6B+LoRA	Val	0.876
	Test	0.895
ChaGLM2-6B+QLoRA	Val	0.875
	Test	0.896
ChaGLM2-6B+EDA	Val	0.874
	Test	0.893
Qwen-7B-Chat	Val	0.878
	Test	0.899
Qwen-7B-Chat+LoRA	Val	0.878
	Test	0.898
Qwen-7B-Chat+QLoRA	Val	0.876
	Test	0.896
Qwen-7B-Chat+EDA	Val	0.879
	Test	0.909

5   Conclusion

In this paper, we propose a new approach to classify diabetic texts. We innovatively propose a framework for model integration, which includes three modules: the combination of large and small models, the large model calling external tools to do data enhancement, and the voting mechanism. We use external tools to expand the number of difficult samples to continuously optimize the model, and then combined with the voting mechanism, the results of multiple model classification will be voted on, and the result with the highest number of votes is taken as the final output using the majority voting strategy. The above framework can effectively reduce the misclassification of some difficult samples due to the uneven distribution of sample data, and effectively improve the accuracy of the model for the classification of special categories of text. The experimental results show that the method can effectively classify medical problems reasonably and achieve a high accuracy rate. Finally, our accuracy rate is 0.92 in the diabetes text categorization task of CHIP 2023 in the test set evaluation, which ranks second in the ranking. In this paper, we proposes a new approach to classifying diabetic texts. A framework for model integration, which includes the following three modules, is innovatively introduced: the combination of large and small models, the large model requiring external tools for data enhancement, and the voting mechanism. External tools are used to expand the number of difficult samples to continuously optimize the model. Combined with the voting mechanism, the results of multiple model classifications will be voted on, and the result with the highest number of votes is taken as the final output using the majority voting strategy. The above framework can effectively reduce the misclassification of some difficult samples due to the uneven distribution of sample data and effectively improve the accuracy of the model for the classification of special categories of text. The experimental results show that the method can successfully classify medical problems reasonably and achieve a high accuracy rate. Overall, the accuracy rate is 0.92 in the diabetes text categorization task of CHIP 2023 in the test set evaluation, which ranks second in the classification.

References

1. Huang, C.-C., Lu, Z.: Community challenges in biomedical text mining over 10 years: success, failure and the future. Brief. Bioinform. **17**(1), 132–144 (2016)
2. Demner-Fushman, D., Chapman, W.W., McDonald, C.J.: What can natural language processing do for clinical decision support? J. Biomed. Inform. **42**(5), 760–772 (2009)
3. Wilcox, A.B., Hripcsak, G.: The role of domain knowledge in automating medical text report classification. J. Am. Med. Inform. Assoc. **10**(4), 330–338 (2003)
4. Suominen, H., et al.: Machine learning to automate the assignment of diagnosis codes to free-text radiology reports: a method description. In: Proceedings of the ICML/UAI/COLT Workshop on Machine Learning for Health-Care Applications (2008)

5. Solt, I., Tikk, D., Gál, V., Kardkovács, Z.T.: Semantic classification of diseases in discharge summaries using a context-aware rule-based classifier. J. Am. Med. Inform. Assoc. **16**(4), 580–584 (2009)

6. Garla, V.N., Brandt, C.: Knowledge-based biomedical word sense disambiguation: an evaluation and application to clinical document classification. J. Am. Med. Inform. Assoc. **20**(5), 882–886 (2013)

7. Garla, V.N., Brandt, C.: Ontology-guided feature engineering for clinical text classification. J. Biomed. Inform. **45**(5), 992–998 (2012)

8. Goodfellow, I., Bengio, Y., Courville, A.: Deep Learning. MIT Press, Cambridge (2016)

9. Valdovinos, R.M., Sánchez, J.S.: Combining multiple classifiers with dynamic weighted voting. In: Corchado, E., Wu, X., Oja, E., Herrero, Á., Baruque, B. (eds.) HAIS 2009. LNCS, vol. 5572, pp. 510–516. Springer, Heidelberg (2009). https://doi.org/10.1007/978-3-642-02319-4_61

10. LeCun, Y., Bottou, L., Bengio, Y., Haffner, P.: Gradient-based learning applied to document recognition. Proc. IEEE **86**(11), 2278–2324 (1998)

11. Kalchbrenner, N., Grefenstette, E., Blunsom, P.: A convolutional neural network for modelling sentences. arXiv preprint arXiv:1404.2188 (2014)

12. Kim, Y.: Convolutional neural networks for sentence classification. arXiv preprint arXiv:1408.5882 (2014)

13. Zaremba, W., Sutskever, I., Vinyals, O.: Recurrent neural network regularization. arXiv preprint arXiv:1409.2329 (2014)

14. Tai, K.S., Socher, R., Manning, C.D.: Improved semantic representations from tree-structured long short-term memory networks. arXiv preprint arXiv:1503.00075 (2015)

15. Hochreiter, S., Schmidhuber, J.: Long short-term memory. Neural Comput. **9**(8), 1735–1780 (1997)

16. Liu, P., Qiu, X., Huang, X.: Recurrent neural network for text classification with multi-task learning. arXiv preprint arXiv:1605.05101 (2016)

17. Devlin, J., Chang, M.-W., Lee, K., Toutanova, K.: BERT: pre-training of deep bidirectional transformers for language understanding. arXiv preprint arXiv:1810.04805 (2018)

18. Chen, X., Sun, Y., Athiwaratkun, B., Cardie, C., Weinberger, K.: Adversarial deep averaging networks for cross-lingual sentiment classification. Trans. Assoc. Comput. Linguist. **6**, 557–570 (2018)

19. Yang, Y., Zhang, M., Chen, W., Zhang, W., Wang, H., Zhang, M.: Adversarial learning for Chinese NER from crowd annotations. In: Proceedings of the AAAI Conference on Artificial Intelligence, vol. 32 (2018)

20. Yasir, M., Wan, J., Liu, S., Hui, S., Xu, M., Hossain, Md.: Coupling of deep learning and remote sensing: a comprehensive systematic literature review. Int. J. Remote Sens. **44**(1), 157–193 (2023)

21. Szegedy, C., et al.: Intriguing properties of neural networks. arXiv preprint arXiv:1312.6199 (2013)

22. Goodfellow, I.J., Shlens, J., Szegedy, C.: Explaining and harnessing adversarial examples. arXiv preprint arXiv:1412.6572 (2014)

23. Miyato, T., Dai, A.M., Goodfellow, I.: Adversarial training methods for semi-supervised text classification. arXiv preprint arXiv:1605.07725 (2016)

24. 李静, 程苋森, 许丽丹, 等.: Name entity recognition based on local adversarial training. J. Sichuan Univ. (Nat. Sci. Ed.) **58**(2), 023003 (2021)

25. Yasunaga, M., Kasai, J., Radev, D.: Robust multilingual part-of-speech tagging via adversarial training. arXiv preprint arXiv:1711.04903 (2017)
26. Zhou, J.T., et al.: Dual adversarial neural transfer for low-resource named entity recognition. In: Proceedings of the 57th Annual Meeting of the Association for Computational Linguistics, pp. 3461–3471 (2019)
27. Wang, X., Aitchison, L., Rudolph, M.: LoRA ensembles for large language model fine-tuning. arXiv preprint arXiv:2310.00035 (2023)
28. Li, C., Farkhoor, H., Liu, R., Yosinski, J.: Measuring the intrinsic dimension of objective landscapes. arXiv preprint arXiv:1804.08838 (2018)
29. Aghajanyan, A., Zettlemoyer, L., Gupta, S.: Intrinsic dimensionality explains the effectiveness of language model fine-tuning. arXiv preprint arXiv:2012.13255 (2020)
30. Yu, A.W., et al.: QANet: combining local convolution with global self-attention for reading comprehension. arXiv preprint arXiv:1804.09541 (2018)
31. Xie, Z., et al.: Data noising as smoothing in neural network language models. arXiv preprint arXiv:1703.02573 (2017)
32. Kobayashi, S.: Contextual augmentation: data augmentation by words with paradigmatic relations. arXiv preprint arXiv:1805.06201 (2018)
33. Wei, J., Zou, K.: EDA: easy data augmentation techniques for boosting performance on text classification tasks. arXiv preprint arXiv:1901.11196 (2019)
34. Schick, T., Schütze, H.: Exploiting cloze questions for few shot text classification and natural language inference. arXiv preprint arXiv:2001.07676 (2020)
35. Reynolds, L., McDonell, K.: Prompt programming for large language models: beyond the few-shot paradigm. In: Extended Abstracts of the 2021 CHI Conference on Human Factors in Computing Systems, pp. 1–7 (2021)
36. Gao, T., Fisch, A., Chen, D.: Making pre-trained language models better few-shot learners. arXiv preprint arXiv:2012.15723 (2020)
37. Liu, X., et al.: GPT understands, too. AI Open (2023)
38. Chen, Z., et al.: Phoenix: democratizing ChatGPT across languages. arXiv preprint arXiv:2304.10453 (2023)
39. Cui, Y., Che, W., Liu, T., Qin, B., Wang, S., Hu, G.: Revisiting pre-trained models for Chinese natural language processing. arXiv preprint arXiv:2004.13922 (2020)
40. Bai, J., et al.: Qwen-VL: a frontier large vision-language model with versatile abilities. arXiv preprint arXiv:2308.12966 (2023)
41. Hu, E.J., et al.: LoRA: low-rank adaptation of large language models. arXiv preprint arXiv:2106.09685 (2021)
42. Dettmers, T., Pagnoni, A., Holtzman, A., Zettlemoyer, L.: QLORA: efficient fine-tuning of quantized LLMs. arXiv preprint arXiv:2305.14314 (2023)
43. Zhuang, Y., Yu, Y., Wang, K., Sun, H., Zhang, C.: ToolQA: a dataset for LLM question answering with external tools. arXiv preprint arXiv:2306.13304 (2023)
44. Yao, J., Zhou, Z., Wang, Q.: Solving math word problem with problem type classification. In: Liu, F., Duan, N., Xu, Q., Hong, Y. (eds.) NLPCC 2023. LNCS, vol. 14304, pp. 123–134. Springer, Cham (2023). https://doi.org/10.1007/978-3-031-44699-3_12

Text Classification Based on Multilingual Back-Translation and Model Ensemble

Jinwang Song, Hongying Zan$^{(\boxtimes)}$, Tao Liu, Kunli Zhang, Xinmeng Ji, and Tingting Cui

School of Computer and Artificial Intelligence, Zhengzhou University, Zhengzhou, China
jwsong@gs.zzu.edu.cn, {iehyzan,ieklzhang}@zzu.edu.cn

Abstract. Pretraining-and-finetuning have demonstrated excellent performance in the field of text classification. However, for downstream tasks, having an ample amount of training data remains crucial. When manually annotated training data is insufficient, a common approach is to perform data augmentation, and back translation using machine translation techniques is a commonly used text augmentation method. However, machine translation may introduce low-quality samples, thereby affecting the effectiveness of text augmentation. In this study, we use pre-trained models to generate sentence embeddings and employ sentence vector similarity comparison to automatically filter back-translated samples, aiming to enhance the quality of back-translation. Combining the ensemble learning approach, we enhance the classification accuracy by integrating multiple sets of diverse models. Our method achieved an accuracy of 90.7 in the 2023 CHIP evaluation task, securing the third-place position.

Keywords: Text Classification · Data Augmentation · Model Ensemble

1 Introduction

Diabetes has emerged as one of the most prevalent global diseases, presenting significant challenges to healthcare resources. Automating the classification of medical consultations for diabetic patients can better guide individuals to seek medical attention and facilitate more efficient allocation of healthcare resources. Patient consultation classification poses a text classification challenge. For specific tasks like classifying diabetes-related questions, constructing a dataset often requires manual annotation, leading to issues such as limited training data, impacting the ultimate performance of pre-trained models on downstream tasks.

Various approaches exist for data processing. Data cleaning involves removing irrelevant noise data to retain valuable information, allowing the model to better fit the data. Data standardization ensures that data from different dimensions adheres to specific rules, eliminating outliers to reduce their impact on model training [1,4,6,11]. Data denoising, a complex aspect of data cleaning, involves distinguishing between essential model information and redundant data. Therefore, data augmentation is employed to enhance both the quantity and quality

© The Author(s), under exclusive license to Springer Nature Singapore Pte Ltd. 2024
H. Xu et al. (Eds.): CHIP 2023, CCIS 2080, pp. 231–241, 2024.
https://doi.org/10.1007/978-981-97-1717-0_21

of data when facing insufficient and low-quality dataset, improving overall effectiveness.

One common Easy Data Augmentation (EDA) method [14] involves back-translating the original dataset to augment it while maintaining semantic consistency [10]. In this evaluation, we adopted a multilingual back-translation method and ensured the quality of translated sentences by calculating the cosine similarity between them. To further enhance predictive performance, we employed model ensemble, combining results from multiple diverse models using a two-stage majority voting approach. In the CHIP 2023 Task 6, focusing on diabetes question classification, our approach achieved the third position in the evaluation results.

Our main contributions include:

1. Multilingual back-translation augmentation (English, Japanese and Korean) of the data, and quality control is performed by computing cosine similarity between sentence vectors generated by the pre-trained semantic embedding model.
2. Model ensemble approach, leveraging two-level voting on predictions from multiple diverse models, resulting in significant improvements compared to individual models.

2   Related Work

2.1   Pre-trained Models

Based on deep learning, text classification algorithms have been a recent research focus. Google introduced BERT, a context-based language model that generates word vectors. BERT is a bidirectional pre-trained language model composed of encoders from the Transformer architecture [13]. When using BERT, one can achieve excellent results by modifying the output layer and fine-tuning the model based on the downstream task [7]. However, the BERT model is trained for longer texts, and its performance on shorter texts is generally less satisfactory. As a result, there have been numerous improved models derived from BERT. For example, RoBERTa [9], ALBERT [8], MacBERT [2]. Including Chinese-based models like BERT-Chinese-wwm [3], and MC-Bert which pre-trained on Chinese biomedical corpus [16], these can be substituted for or better address downstream tasks compared to the original BERT.

2.2   Text Classification

Text classification task is one of the most common tasks in natural language processing. RoBERTa can achieve better performance in text classification tasks through fine-tuning for specific domains or tasks. ALBERT is also suitable for text classification tasks, and its streamlined model structure is particularly useful in resource-constrained environments. BERT-Chinese-wwm is a BERT model pre-trained on a Chinese corpus, taking into consideration the characteristics of the Chinese language and incorporating processing methods like WordPiece tokenization tailored for Chinese. When used for Chinese text classification tasks, BERT-Chinese-wwm can adapt to different domains or specific task requirements through fine-tuning. Although pre-trained models like RoBERTa, ALBERT, MacBERT, BERT-Chinese-wwm perform well in tasks such as text classification, they also have some drawbacks and limitations. RoBERTa, despite optimizations over the original BERT model, still requires substantial computing resources for training and fine-tuning. ALBERT's transfer learning effectiveness may be constrained when there is significant dissimilarity between the source and target domains. MacBERT's performance might be constrained by the quality and quantity of pre-training data. In specific tasks, MacBERT's performance may not differ significantly from that of general pre-trained models. BERT-Chinese-wwm may face challenges in handling certain fine-grained tasks in Chinese, such as word segmentation and entity recognition. The uneven distribution of data is a significant characteristic of the CHIP 2023 Task Six on diabetes problem classification. Integrating multiple models is better suited to capture the diversity within the data. In this study, we integrated MacBERT and RoBERTa-Base and RoBERTa-Large, leveraging the strengths of MacBERT and RoBERTa. By combining predictions from multiple models, we aimed to enhance overall performance while reducing reliance on individual models, thereby improving the overall system's robustness.

3   Methods

3.1   Multilingual Back-Translation

For the choice of the Easy Data Augmentation (EDA) method, we opted for back-translation. A well-executed back-translation can modify vocabulary, syntax, word order, length, and other aspects of a sentence while preserving the overall semantics, thereby expanding the training sample. The conventional approach to back-translation involves single-language back-translation [12], such as Chinese → Intermediate language → Chinese, resulting in a maximum doubling of the training set. We employed a multilingual back-translation approach, translating from Chinese → (Intermediate language 1, Intermediate language 2, Intermediate language 3... Intermediate language N) → Chinese, to achieve a more robust augmentation effect.

Nevertheless, back-translation comes with its challenges. Due to the limitations of machine translation, there may be instances of low-quality translations that deviate from the original sentence's meaning, particularly for shorter and more colloquial texts. The occurrence of low-quality samples may be more pronounced In the case of multilingual back-translation. To address this and enhance the quality of back-translation, we implemented a filtering method using sentence vector similarity comparison. This approach involves calculating the similarity between sentence vectors before and after back-translation, allowing us to assess the quality of the translation and filter out low-quality samples. As the Fig. 1 shows.

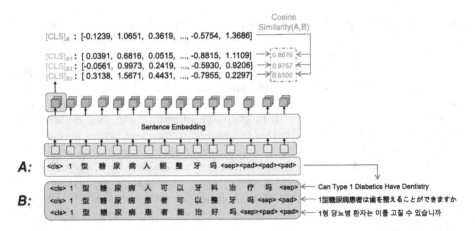

Fig. 1. Back translation process

A represents the original text, and B represents the back-translated text. Sentence vectors are generated by a pre-trained embedding model, using the last hidden state of the first token in the input (i.e., [CLS]) as the sentence representation. Then calculate the cosine similarity between A and B. At the same time a threshold is set, back-translation samples with a cosine similarity less than the threshold are discarded.

3.2 Model Ensemble

We fine-tuned multiple text classification models as sub-models, and the sub-models performed Majority Voting to determine the final result. According to the formula for ensemble learning: representing the predicted output of h_i on sample x as an N-dimensional vector $(h_i^1(x); h_i^2(x); ...,h_i^N(x))$ where $h_i^j(x)$ is the output of h_i for class label c_i. We employed a relative majority voting method as Eq. 1.

$$H(x) = C_{arg\,max\,\sum_{i=1}^{T} h_x^j(x)} \tag{1}$$

The better the individual learner's accuracy and diversity, the more effective the ensemble. After fusion, better results are achieved [17], and we create diverse models from different perspectives.

Data: We trained sub-models using different datasets, with some using the unmodified original training set and others using the training set augmented through back-translation.

Input: Adversarial training was applied to some sub-models by perturbing the Embedding layer during fine-tuning using the Fast Gradient Method (FGM).

Hyperparameters/Settings: Various batch sizes and learning rates were experimented with for sub-models. Different learning rates were applied to the pre-trained layer and the classification layer. Dropout layers in the pre-training layer were disabled in some sub-models.

Output Layer: For the output of pre-trained models, different approaches were explored. One involved individually inputting the last layer's [CLS] token into an MLP as a classifier. Another method used LSTM, BiLSTM, and AttentionPooling as pooling layers to extract all hidden states from the final layer's output of the pre-trained model. As the Fig. 2 shows.

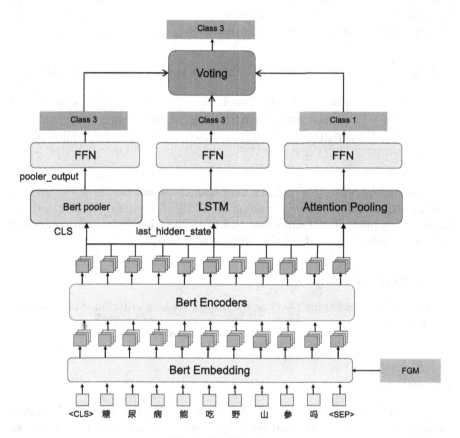

Fig. 2. Model structure

4   Experiment

4.1   Dataset

The dataset is derived from the dataset provided by the CHIP 2023 task. The dataset consists of Chinese diabetes-related questions categorized into six classes, including diagnosis, treatment, common knowledge, healthy lifestyle, epidemiology, and others. For the specific back-translation method, the Baidu General Text Translation API was employed. It translated 6,000 Chinese sentences from the original training set into English, Japanese, and Korean. Moreover, these translations were independently back-translated into Chinese from English, Japanese, and Korean, resulting in an initial set of 18,000 back-translated samples. We utilized the open-source bge-large-zh-v1.5 as the embedding model [5,15] and set the similarity threshold to 0.7. Comparing the cosine similarity between each original sample and its corresponding back-translated sample, we filtered out low-quality back-translated samples with a similarity less than 0.7. The entire set was then deduplicated. Table 1 provides a comparison of the training set before and after back-translation.

Table 1. Comparison of number of training set samples and label distribution.

Train set	Total	Class 0	Class 1	Class 2	Class 3	Class 4	Class 5
Original	6000	527	1702	1226	599	1501	445
Augmentation	19615	1690	5441	4098	1815	5090	1481

After incorporating the filtered back-translated samples into the original training set, a final augmented training set of 19615 samples was obtained. No changes were made to the validation and test data; the original validation and test sets were used throughout the experimental process.

4.2 Evaluation Index

The task employs accuracy (Acc) as the overall ranking criterion. The quation 2 is as follows.

$$Accuracy = \frac{Predicted}{Total} \tag{2}$$

4.3 Setting

Using the Adam optimizer with default parameters. For the base model, a tiered learning rate was employed, and the sub-models used batch sizes of 32, 64, 96, and 128. For the large model, sub-models were experimented with batch sizes of 32, 48, 64, and 72. Learning rates were experimented with, specifically, 1e−5, 2e−5, 3e−5, and 4e−5 for the layers, and for the classification layer, learning rates of 2e−5, 4e−5, 5e−5, and 1e−4 were attempted. The number of epochs was set to 10, and the validation set accuracy was tested after each epoch. Save the model weights of the epoch with the highest validation set score. In a single round of experimentation, nine different models were designed, grouped into three sets. Within each set, Majority Voting was performed to determine the final result. The results within each group were subjected to a second round of Majority Voting. Additionally, adversarial training using the Fast Gradient Method was applied to perturb the embedding layer for some sub-models.

4.4   Result and Analysis

Performance Comparison of Different Pre-trained Models. To compare the performance of pre-trained models, we selected the models with superior performance. In the evaluation task on the original dataset, dev_acc represents the accuracy on the validation set, and test_acc represents the accuracy on the test set after submission. We experimented with five Chinese pre-trained models, and the results are shown in Table 2.

Table 2. Performance Disparities Among Different Pre-trained Models.

Model	dev_acc	test_acc
bert-base-chinese	85.6	87.8
chinese_roberta_wwm_ext	86.3	88.4
chinese_roberta_wwm_large_ext	87.7	88.9
chinese-macbert-large	87.5	–
mc_bert_base	85.5	–

Through testing five pre-trained models, it is evident that in terms of model size the performance of large-sized pre-trained models is superior to that of base-sized pre-trained models. This is attributed to the larger network structure and greater number of parameters in the large model. In terms of model types, RoBERTa exhibits the best performance, followed by MacBERT, both of which outperform BERT and MC_BERT. This might be attributed to the fact that RoBERTa and MacBERT adopt more effective pre-training strategies and longer pre-training processes, leading to better performance in downstream tasks compared to the original BERT. In conclusion, through the comparison of pre-trained model performances, we selected RoBERTa as the best-performing model and MacBERT as the secondary model for subsequent experiments.

Table 3. Performance of the model before and after training set back-translation augmentation

dataset	model	250 steps	500steps	750 steps	1000 steps
Original	bert-base-chinese	0.843	0.860	0.851	0.857
	chinese_roberta_wwm_ext	0.85	0.860	0.849	0.856
	chinese-macbert-base	0.849	0.859	0.855	0.859
Augmentation	bert-base-chinese	0.837	0.862	0.866	0.866
	chinese_roberta_wwm_ext	0.845	0.858	0.870	0.865
	chinese-macbert-base	0.849	0.852	0.862	0.863

Impact of Training Set on Experimental Results. Table 3 presents the impact of the dataset before and after augmentation on the model's performance through comparative experiments.

Under identical conditions, we compared the accuracy of the original validation set during the fine-tuning process across three pre-trained models based on the number of update steps. The experiment maintained consistent hyperparameters, and the random seed was set to 2. The experimental results reveal that during fine-tuning with the original training set, the model outperforms the augmented dataset group before 500 steps, reaching the highest validation set accuracy around 500 steps. However, after 500 steps, the validation set accuracy starts to decline, indicating the occurrence of overfitting. During fine-tuning with the augmented training set, the model's accuracy steadily increases within the first 1000 steps, ultimately surpassing the highest dev_acc achieved by the fine-tuning group with the original dataset. Moreover, basically no overfitting phenomenon is observed. This suggests that after training set augmentation, the sample space is expanded, and imparting the model with greater generalization.

Impact of Similarity Threshold on Model Performance. We explored the accuracy of the model under different similarity threshold on three pre-trained models using a discard threshold of 0.0 (i.e., all back-translated samples were used), 0.7(ours), 0.85 respectively, and the original training set as a baseline, using a filter to smooth the data and plotting line graphs. As the Fig. 3 shows.

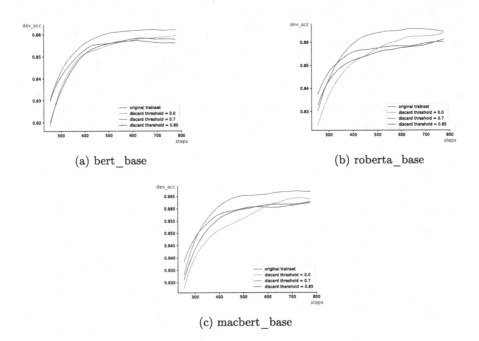

(a) bert_base   (b) roberta_base

(c) macbert_base

Fig. 3. Models performance under different thresholds

It can be seen that the model performs best with the setting threshold=0.7. When decreasing threshold further to 0, all back-translation samples are added to the training set without discarding, resulting in a decrease in accuracy, which shows the detrimental effect of low-quality back-translation samples and proves the necessity of quality control for back-translation. Meanwhile, increasing threshold to 0.85 and discarding more low-similarity samples also causes a decrease in accuracy, which in some cases is even lower than the baseline. This may be due to the fact that the higher similarity threshold causes the added back-translated samples to be too close to the original texts, thus failing to effectively increase the feature space of the training set. The experiments show that choosing a good threshold is important. An appropriate threshold can avoid the low-quality texts brought by back-translation while retaining samples with diversity.

Impact of Model Ensemble on Experimental Results. For model ensemble, as Table 4 a simple majority voting was conducted for every three sets of sub-models. In cases where there was no majority within a group (i.e., all three sub-models predicted differently), the result of the sub-model with the highest validation set accuracy was selected.

Table 4. Comparison of accuracy before and after model ensemble.

Pre-trained model	Classification layer	Dataset	Dev_acc	Test_acc(after voting)
roberta_large	MLP	Original	87.8	89.3	90.5
roberta_large	BiLSTM	Original	87.3	
roberta_base	LSTM	Original	86.3	
roberta_large+FGM	MLP	Augmentation	88.1	90.0
roberta_large	BiLSTM	Original	87.7	
roberta_large	MLP	Augmentation	87.1	
roberta_large	Attention Polling	Original	87.7	89.6
roberta_large+FGM	BiLSTM	Augmentation	87.3	
macbert_large+FGM	MLP	Augmentation	87.5	

It can be observed that after combining the results of the sub-models, the accuracy improved on the basis of the highest accuracy achieved by the individual sub-models. This indicates that the sub-models designed have some diversity, ensuring the effectiveness of model ensemble. For the ensemble method, we utilized a two-level voting approach. Compared to the single-level voting method where all sub-models directly vote, we believe that the two-level voting method makes more comprehensive use of the results from all sub-models, bringing greater uncertainty but a higher upper bound.

5   Conclusion

In addressing the text classification diabetes question, we employed multi-language back-translation with similarity comparison to augment the training set. Leveraging multiple pre-trained models as a foundation, we fine-tuned several diverse sub-models and integrate their predictions. Our experiments on the Chinese Diabetes Question Classification Task in CHIP 2023 show that our approach elevates the test set results to 90.7, demonstrating a significant impact of model ensemble on classification outcomes.

Acknowledgements. This research was supported by the National Natural Science Foundation of China (Grant No. 62006211), the key research and development and promotion project of Henan Provincial Department of Science and Technology in 2023 (232102211041), Science and technology research project of Henan Provincial science and Technology Department in 2023(232102211033) and Science and Technology Innovation 2030-"New Generation of Artificial Intelligence" Major Project under Grant No. 2021ZD0111000. We want to acknowledge the valuable data support provided by SEMRC, CVDEMRC, and CMeIE. We would like to thank the anonymous reviewers for their valuable comments and suggestions on the improvement of this paper.

References

1. Clark, E., Araki, K.: Text normalization in social media: progress, problems and applications for a pre-processing system of casual English. Procedia Soc. Behav. Sci. **27**, 2–11 (2011)
2. Cui, Y., Che, W., Liu, T., Qin, B., Wang, S., Hu, G.: Revisiting pre-trained models for Chinese natural language processing. In: Findings of the Association for Computational Linguistics: EMNLP 2020, pp. 657–668 (2020)
3. Cui, Y., Che, W., Liu, T., Qin, B., Yang, Z.: Pre-training with whole word masking for Chinese bert. IEEE/ACM Trans. Audio Speech Lang. Process. **29**, 3504–3514 (2021)
4. Desai, N., Narvekar, M.: Normalization of noisy text data. Procedia Comput. Sci. **45**, 127–132 (2015)
5. Dong, X., Yu, Z., Cao, W., Shi, Y., Ma, Q.: A survey on ensemble learning. Front. Comput. Sci. **14**, 241–258 (2020)
6. Esnaola, L., Tessore, J.P., Ramón, H., Russo, C.: Effectiveness of preprocessing techniques over social media texts for the improvement of machine learning based classifiers. In: 2019 XLV Latin American Computing Conference (CLEI), pp. 1–10. IEEE (2019)
7. Kenton, J.D.M.W.C., Toutanova, L.K.: Bert: pre-training of deep bidirectional transformers for language understanding. In: Proceedings of the NAACL-HLT, pp. 4171–4186 (2019)
8. Lan, Z., Chen, M., Goodman, S., Gimpel, K., Sharma, P., Soricut, R.: Albert: a lite bert for self-supervised learning of language representations (2020)
9. Liu, Y., et al.: Roberta: a robustly optimized bert pretraining approach (2019)
10. Ma, J., Li, L.: Data augmentation for Chinese text classification using back-translation. J. Phys.: Conf. Ser. **1651**, 012039. IOP Publishing (2020)

11. Pradha, S., Halgamuge, M.N., Vinh, N.T.Q.: Effective text data preprocessing technique for sentiment analysis in social media data. In: 2019 11th International Conference on Knowledge and Systems Engineering (KSE), pp. 1–8. IEEE (2019)
12. Sennrich, R., Haddow, B., Birch, A.: Improving neural machine translation models with monolingual data. In: Proceedings of the 54th Annual Meeting of the Association for Computational Linguistics (Volume 1: Long Papers), pp. 86–96 (2016)
13. Vaswani, A., et al.: Attention is all you need. Adv. Neural Inf. Process. Syst. **30** (2017)
14. Wei, J., Zou, K.: EDA: easy data augmentation techniques for boosting performance on text classification tasks. In: Proceedings of the 2019 Conference on Empirical Methods in Natural Language Processing and the 9th International Joint Conference on Natural Language Processing (EMNLP-IJCNLP), pp. 6382–6388 (2019)
15. Xiao, S., Liu, Z., Zhang, P., Muennighoff, N.: C-Pack: packaged resources to advance general Chinese embedding (2023)
16. Zhang, N., Jia, Q., Yin, K., Dong, L., Gao, F., Hua, N.: Conceptualized representation learning for Chinese biomedical text mining (2020)
17. Zhou, Z.H.: Ensemble Methods: Foundations and Algorithms. CRC Press, Boca Raton (2012)

Author Index

© The Editor(s) (if applicable) and The Author(s), under exclusive license
to Springer Nature Singapore Pte Ltd. 2024
H. Xu et al. (Eds.): CHIP 2023, CCIS 2080, pp. 243–244, 2024.
https://doi.org/10.1007/978-981-97-1717-0

Printed in the United States
by Baker & Taylor Publisher Services